stand in your TRUTH

SEVEN SACRED TRUTHS TO LIVING A DIVINELY GUIDED LIFE

SUZY SCHAAK

stand in your TRUTH

SEVEN SACRED TRUTHS TO LIVING
A DIVINELY GUIDED LIFE

Edited by George Verongos

Cover art: *After the Storm* by Suzy Schaak

ISBN: 979-8-218-29954-5

About the Cover

The imagery in *After The Storm* represents the emotional and spiritual struggles we, in our humanity, manage throughout our lives. Think of these struggles like a cloud of congestion held within the body. As we remember our innate wisdom and Stand In Our Truth, the clouds begin to clear, and the sky opens up, illuminating this blessed truth—we are perfect, Divine, sacred beings, living in the vastness of Divine Love.

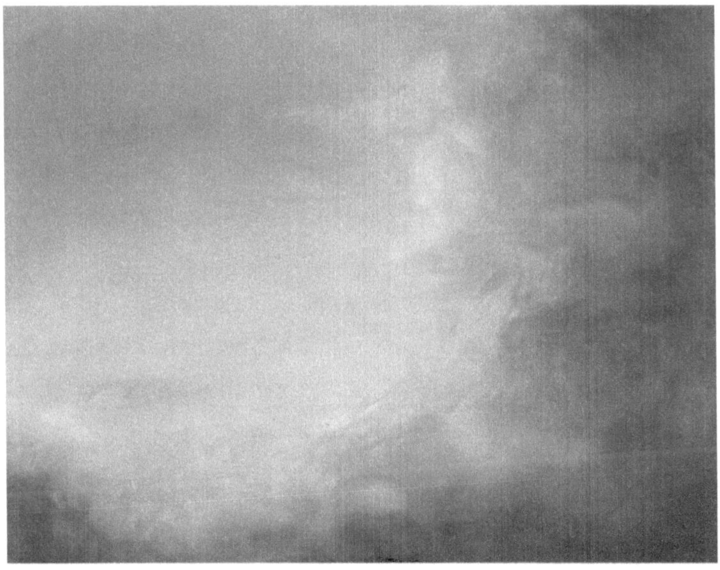

To purchase a print of *After The Storm* or other pieces by Suzy, scan the QR code or visit the link.

https://www.etsy.com/shop/SuzySchaak

About the Author

Suzy Schaak is a clairvoyant healer and a channel for your guides, angels, and master healers. In her work, she shares wisdom revealed by Divine realms to offer greater insight and lasting well-being. Suzy started on the path to mastery in the healing arts in 2001 and has extensive experience in hands-on healing and clairvoyant reading. As a passionate yogini, E-RYT 500, and meditation instructor, Suzy has worked with thousands of students. She describes herself as being in the business of transformation, whether it be through her healing sessions, yoga and meditation classes, destination retreats, or her signature 200-Hr Yoga Studies & Teacher Training Program. Please visit Suzy's website to book a healing session and for further information.

www.suzyschaakyoga.com

Yoga & Meditation

I have recorded chapter-specific introduction, yoga, and meditation videos to further deepen your exploration of each Sacred Truth and to assist in awakening and healing physically, emotionally, and spiritually. The yoga & meditation component of this book is about listening to the wisdom of your body and your breath to guide you through stillness and movement. The yoga sequences are designed for everyone to participate in a way that brings you to a place of gentle awareness, surrendering, transformation, and healing. You are encouraged to explore the movements in a way that serves you best—with grace and nurturing for your sweet, beautiful body. **Please check with your healthcare provider if you have any pre-existing conditions or injuries to confirm that participating in this activity is safe.**

Sign up using the link at the end of each chapter.

In Humble Gratitude...

To my Fab Five

Joe—the moment I met you, I felt the most profound soul connection. You have supported me unconditionally through each twist and turn in my life. From walking alongside me as my dad was dying to showing me grace and patience over the last three years while I pulled back from the world to grieve and write. You have always allowed me the time, space, and encouragement to grow into who I am today. I love you truly, madly, deeply.

Sister Love—Madeline, Lily, and Charlotte—the sun rises and sets around the three of you. Your wise souls have taught me so much over the years. Each of you is so unique and yet meld so beautifully together as sisters and best friends. It has been an honor to be your mom, and as you have grown into women, I have the joy of also being your friend. My heart is full. I love you. I love you. I love you cause I do.

To my mom, Mary—Your open mind, curiosity, support, and love have continually guided me forward. I have always felt that I can share anything with you. You are my role model as a strong, independent, and nurturing woman—not only for myself but also for your beautiful granddaughters. I love you unconditionally! Oh—and besides RBG, I don't know another 84-year-old woman who can hold a plank pose for an entire minute!

My sweet, sweet Dad—I have felt your presence so strongly through the writing of this book. The biggest lessons I learned from you are to walk humbly through this world, recognize and appreciate the goodness all around me, and love fearlessly. With all my heart, I love you, Dad.

Pat & Dick Schaak—I could not have asked for more amazing in-laws. Pat, I love you for all of your big open-armed hugs followed by a "Hi, Suz" and joyful family times centered around Sunday dinners. Dick, since my dad passed, you have stepped in and supported me with such kind words and encouragement. You have filled a place in my heart with your fatherly love.

Lynnie Lou—There are no words to describe the joy and laughter you have brought into my life. Your friendship feels like a miracle that blessed me when I so badly needed a friend. It is a celebration every time you come home to visit. I'm looking forward to our next thigh master/ping-pong extravaganza. Love you! Love you! Love you!

Carol Bruess—You have been the greatest cheerleader throughout this entire process. Your guidance and enthusiasm have meant the world to me. With all the love in my heart, thank you!

Lisa Proctor Hawkins—From the day you invited me to tea, throughout all of our Monday night date nights after yoga, until now, you have continually encouraged me to acknowledge my strength and progress, challenge what I thought was possible, and move forward into the unknown. I love you, sweet lady!

Lisa Reiner—Joy! Joy! Joy! That is how I think of you. You are the embodiment of pure Mama Love! As my perfect client, this book was written with you continually in my heart.

Leo—We have walked quite a journey together. Over the past three years, you continually demonstrate what is possible through your enthusiasm for life and listening to your inner guidance. I couldn't love you more!

BT—so much gratitude for your Divine Loving Wisdom as my mentor and dear friend.

I dedicate this book in loving memory to my dad and Tyler.

Contents

Introduction

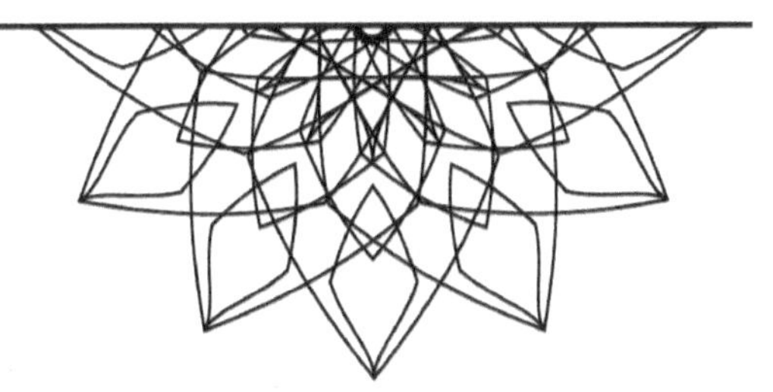

In the spring and summer of 2020, I was in the middle of what I would call *the perfect storm.* As the entire world was walking blindly through a global pandemic, I was recovering from the wrath of Lyme disease and trying to find my footing after one of the most traumatic experiences of my life. In May of 2020, I also chose to walk away from my successful yoga business that I had grown for more than ten years and step into an abyss of isolation, trying to heal—both emotionally and physically—and find myself again. During this time of silence, I have never felt so lost and, strangely, so cradled in light. I pulled myself from the world, creating a self-made cocoon where I journaled, meditated, and spent countless hours walking through the forest. I knew this was a time of rebirth—not just for me but for the entire world.

My time in silence allowed me to bring forward *Stand In Your Truth.* I chose to write this book because the phrase "*Stand In Your Truth*" is an ever-present reminder and guide for me, one urging me to live in alignment with Spirit and love.

While our human form may seem solid, we are all energetic beings. When our energetic channels are in alignment, we feel joyful, creative, powerful, expressive, intuitive, and grounded. It is in these moments we literally "stand" in our truth. But what can you do when a challenging event, loss, or fear knocks you off your axis?

The Seven Sacred Truths—revealed one by one in chapters one through seven—are a roadmap to living in synchronicity. These concepts are true no matter your religious affiliation or upbringing. When we collaborate with Spirit, all resistance fades away, we raise our vibration, and we find a life saturated with ease, joy, and abundance.

As a clairvoyant healer, I receive information from Divine Realms in the form of light, words, an internal impression, or inner knowingness, and images—almost like a movie screen in my mind showing me snapshots of information. This guidance comes from many sources. In the healing sessions, I am communicating with Divine Mother, Yeshua, a person's Soul, their angels, guides, or loved ones who have passed on. Oftentimes, it is a combination of all the above.

I have most recently been channeling the wisdom of Divine Mother. Think of Divine Mother as Mother God, Mother Earth, or Gaia; I like to call her Mama Love. When she appears in my healing sessions, the room fills with the colors of dawn as she ushers in a sacred nurturing Light of compassion and love. Divine Mother's message is unwavering, "We are love." Her request is that we stand in this truth to raise our individual vibration, thus elevating the vibration of our planet. As I sat in hours of meditation to figure out how to get her message out, the content for *Stand In Your Truth* emerged.

To stand in one's truth is to understand that our *human* experiences and *Spiritual* experiences are not separate. Our higher self is always expressing itself through the wisdom of our bodies. Our job is to pause and listen. I describe Seven Sacred Truths in this book. These truths align with the body's energy centers, called chakras. The chakras are important because they bridge our Spiritual experience and life force into our physical body. Integrating these truths is like learning a new language between your body and Spirit. The goal of this book is to introduce you to this language so you have a constant, fluent conversation between the two.

We are in unprecedented times: social and political upheaval, a climate crisis, and unparalleled loneliness. *Stand In Your Truth* is a guide and a resource to help people not only survive but thrive in this physical world. This book is a source of hope, revealing that you can make a difference on our beautiful planet simply by going inward, listening to the voice of your Divine Inner Wisdom, and living your life in alignment with love.

My Story

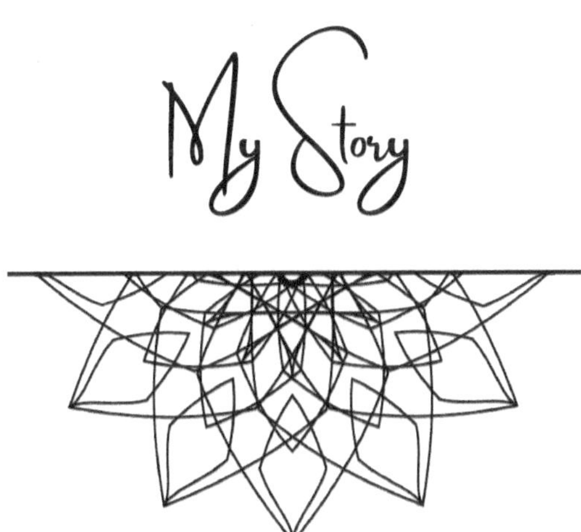

"And above all, watch with glittering eyes the whole world around you because the greatest secrets are always hidden in the most unlikely places. Those who don't believe in magic will never find it." –Roald Dahl

When I was a little girl, my favorite television show was reruns of *I Dream Of Jeannie*. I loved it so much that my mom found some pink Jeannie pajamas just like the ones Barbara Eden wore in the show. I felt beyond special because they were shipped all the way from Las Vegas (don't judge) to my home in Minnesota. These pajamas were not some cheap, sad, flammable nylon costume. Instead, this two-piece little number was made of layers and layers of pure pink chiffon heaven, designed to make any little girl feel like a 2,000-year-old magical genie.

The day they arrived, I ran straight upstairs and put on my bewitching pink ensemble. To complete this magical look, I threw my hair in a high ponytail, popped a styrofoam cup on my head, poked a hole through the top, and pulled my ponytail through the hole. With my outfit complete, I looked and felt fabulous!

I loved this show and my outfit with such intensity because I truly believed in magic and miracles. I spent hours focusing on objects in my room, trying to make them move with the power of my will and sharp focus. I attempted to send and receive thoughts to and from people. I just knew that if I focused long enough, I could blink myself out of my room and into another reality. Something in me knew there was more than what the eyes can see, the ears can hear, and the hands can touch—something beyond our five senses. I didn't know the words for it then, but I was certain there was more than how things appeared on the surface.

Let's just say the practice time in my bedroom was good training because I continue to believe in magic and miracles. As I got a little older, I was able to put a language to it because I began to have experiences that did indeed cross over the five senses. These experiences were given to me one by one, allowing me to integrate and understand this new communication of Divine Wisdom.

The first experience I had was when I was about ten years old. One of my favorite things to do as a little girl was to bundle up in my snowsuit, go outside on a clear winter's night, and lie like a snow angel while looking up at the stars. There was a hush that the deep snow provided, highlighting a mystical feeling from the stillness and silence of winter.

On this particular night of stargazing, I was looking over at my neighbor's house. A few days prior, the husband who lived there had been struck by a car while out for a jog. Tragically, he did not survive the accident. That night, I noticed many cars in the driveway because his family and friends were gathering at their house. I remember wondering how they were feeling because it was such a sudden and sad event. As I was observing the house, a breathtaking circle of light descended over the rooftop. I received my first Divine Message while trying to make sense of what I was seeing. This internal voice said, "The angels are accompanying the spirit of your neighbor, blessing him with the gift of seeing and feeling his family's love." What a tender and sacred moment I was able to witness! I remember thinking, "Well, of course, this sort of thing happens."

As I entered my early teen years, I began to hear this Divine Inner Voice more regularly. This voice still addresses me as *"My Child"* and has become a continual internal dialogue throughout my life. It is filled with compassion and unbiased loving wisdom and is ever-present without fail. The only time I do not hear it is when I step into the distractions of earthly life and do not take the time to be still and listen.

In high school, I had my first vision of a Soul that had crossed over. I woke up early in the morning, and rather than just sparkles of light; I saw an apparition of a young man in a red basketball uniform sitting on my dresser. With elbows resting on his knees and head in his hands, he looked much like the statue of *The Thinker*. He gently observed me as one would watch a baby sleep. I didn't feel afraid. He wanted nothing from me but to simply let me know he was there. The beauty in this moment is that we had a soul exchange—my soul was witnessing his purest unconditional love as he was witnessing mine. We could see beyond what a thinking mind tells us what love is all about. This experience was profoundly serene. He had the peacefulness of an angel sitting in my room, watching over and protecting me. I prayed for the angels to look after him. I then laid back down and fell asleep. When I awoke again, he was gone.

In my college years, all went silent. I was too busy with the distractions of new friends, new experiences, and school. It wasn't until after the birth of my first daughter that my gift returned. It did so in a way that there was no possibility of missing it. Shortly after her birth, I began to receive visitations from the other side, dropping in nearly every night, regardless of my location.

These experiences always began with me feeling very hot. It was this heat that woke me up. I could feel a subtle presence around me. Then, out of the darkness, I would see a vibration of light, very much like a neon sign. The light would slowly vibrate and form an image. My first vision was of a massive "third eye" that filled the entire ceiling. I have to say, it was a bit startling and also pretty extraordinary at the same time. Not knowing what else to do, I prayed for protection. My Divine Wisdom told me this image was a symbol of my reawakening. In my wildest dreams, I could never have imagined what I would be awakening into.

The next night, I had the same sensation. Something felt hot on my face, and the vibrating light began. This time, the vision was of a John Wayne type of character, equal in size to the large third eye. He was riding a rocking horse, wildly cackling while tossing his head back. The image abruptly became deadly serious, and it gazed ominously at my sleeping hubby, Joe. The image pulled out a large gun and aimed it directly at Joe's head. My heart was beating a mile a minute, wondering if it could actually harm us. I remember thinking, *How in the world do I protect Joe or myself from whatever this is?* I shook Joe awake and asked, "Do you see that??" He looked at me and asked, "See what?" "THAT! On the ceiling!!" His response was a simple "No." He rolled back over and went to sleep. I prayed very fast, "Please, please, please, surround Joe and me with light. Protect us from whatever *this* is." As quickly as John Wayne arrived, he faded away while I prayed.

These unusual experiences happened night after night for a couple of years. Some images were pleasant, but most of the time, they morphed into some sort of crazy-looking creature, like flying gargoyles or other entities with biting teeth. During this time, I met with my priest, healers, intuitives—truly anyone who may be able to help me make sense of it. My priest said that he hears stories like this more than one would think. He suggested that I ignore it and don't give it any attention. I thought, *If you had a flying, biting gargoyle coming at you every night, explain how you would ignore that.* The healers and intuitives I spoke with didn't seem to have any great answers either. What I found that always seemed to dissolve or neutralize the images was the Light I brought in while praying for protection during the experience.

After not receiving any true concrete answers, I eventually went deep into conversation with my inner voice. The response I received was that these visions are Spirits in what I call "The In-Between," meaning they are souls who have crossed over and have chosen not to ascend to Heaven and instead remained in the earthly realm. It could be because they don't know where they are due to a sudden or traumatic death, or they have chosen to stay around due to attachments to loved ones, religious beliefs, etc. They came to visit me because I could see them. And they came in that form so that I would pay attention to them. They simply didn't know how to change their circumstances, and the Light from prayer gave them comfort.

My Divine Wisdom told me to guide them to this light, and Spirit will take it from there. So after two years of visitations, I only needed to speak to these souls with compassion and love, encouraging them to "go to the light." I reassured them that the Light is the purest love they will ever know, and that their loved ones on earth would feel a sense of ease once they ascend. On the first night I tried this, my neon visitors turned into a cloud of light that dissolved into a mist and ascended right before my eyes. It looked almost like a vacuum sucked up the light, and off they went. I did this night after night for several months. As I became more fluent with this, I requested they no longer visit me in the middle of the night. I made a declaration that my office hours are daytime only.

In my late thirties, I now had three beautiful girls. My clairvoyant gifts were strong but unfocused. At this time, I began to feel like I needed to serve a bigger purpose. After many years as a wardrobe stylist in the film and fashion show industries, my career no longer seemed to fulfill me. I was recently yoga certified and chose to leave my career as a stylist to open a yoga studio. I spent a year creating a business plan and meeting with anyone and everyone who had experience with small business operations and yoga studio ownership. I took my earnings from my last film job and put down a deposit on a studio space. In this space, there was a wellness room that needed a practitioner. I was desperately trying to rent it out. After almost a year of searching, I received a nudge from Divine Wisdom saying, "That space is for you, silly! It's time for you to step into your healing ministry."

At this time, I had no formal training in the healing arts but had done some sessions with friends that went really well. I purposely chose not to get formal training because I just knew that my internal wisdom would guide me along this path. I felt training with someone else, using a different method, would disrupt the beautiful flow of light and communication I had already established. Shortly after practicing with some friends, I began seeing clients from the studio. I found such ease and joy in these early sessions. It was as if I had learned to speak a new language fluently, and it felt like I had been doing this work for lifetimes.

Prologue

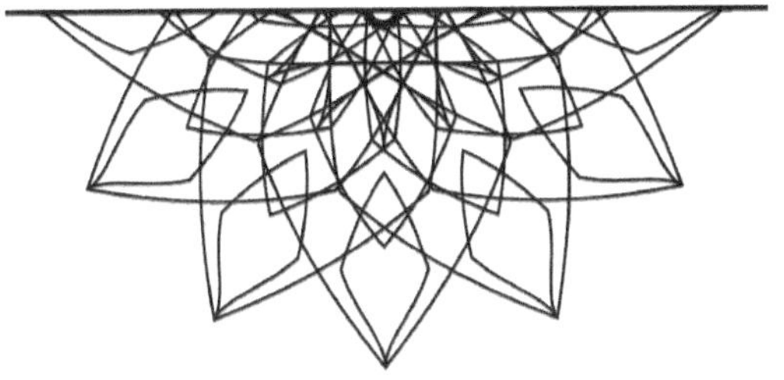

Reflecting on my journey, it truly began when I first heard my internal voice. My heart knew it was the voice of Yeshua—the Hebrew name for Jesus. Rather than seeing Yeshua through the lens and constructs of organized Western religion, I saw Yeshua as a Universal Love that belongs to everyone—not just those who subscribe to a particular belief system. Yeshua communicates through the heart and not necessarily through words but through impressions filled with intense compassion, humility, humor, and love.

The understanding I received in my conversations with Yeshua is that he came into human form to teach and show us what it means to stand in our truth at all times and to live in alignment by fully integrating love, compassion, and joy into our human experience. And through his pure alignment to Spirit, he could manifest miracles because he was never separate from his Source. *That* was his most important message. When we align and co-create with Spirit, we, too, can manifest miracles and have a constant, continuous flow of communication and union with Spirit through our souls.

Many people were afraid of this message. They couldn't understand his unyielding sense of joy and peacefulness. He showed up in this world and deconstructed all of the rules. Because when you live in truth, there are no rules. You are guided by Spirit because you are Spirit. You are guided entirely by love because you are love. When I say that, I don't mean love as an emotion or action, I mean it as the pure essence of your *beingness*. Love is who you are. It is who I am. It is who Yeshua is.

As I said, Yeshua has been communicating with me for most of my life. I know Yeshua to be perfection. I could describe him with many adjectives—love, joy, beauty—but his essence is perfection. And what Yeshua and Divine Mother want us to know is that we are also perfect. We just need to find our way back to the simplicity of that truth. We are love. And there is nothing more to it. Rules and structure are not required if you live in this truth because you don't want to be anything but love. You don't live in a lower vibration that wants to harm, control, or be afraid. It's just like you are cradled and wrapped in this knowingness that *"all is well"* at all times—no matter the circumstance. Yeshua was trying to show us that by living in alignment, we *know* Heaven is not someplace up in the clouds. Heaven lives within us, and it becomes us.

I want to speak for a minute about Divine Mother. As I said, Divine Mother shows up as Mother God, Mother Earth, the feminine aspect of Spirit. She came into human form as Mary, the mother of Yeshua. Her role was to birth the Light of Christ—meaning the Light of pure compassion and love—into the world. In the Buddhist tradition, this Light is called Vairochana. As I say this, it is important to know that what I am expressing has nothing to do with religion or separation. This message is all-inclusive. There is but one Spirit that resides within every living thing—no matter what name you give it. The

20

essence of Spirit is unconditional love. The life of Yeshua and Divine Mother was to show how expansive, all-inclusive, all-loving, and all-nurturing life can be if we live in this truth of unconditional love.

This book is entitled *Stand In Your Truth,* and I have written about the sacred truths as a guide—not as a rule book—but as a guide to remembering your birthright. And that birthright and truth is that you are love, that I am love, that we are love, that we are one, that we are Spirit living a human experience. And it's time for us to remember who we are and live with the compassion that Yeshua and Divine Mother came to show us.

I hope you enjoy the book because, within each chapter, I am offering experiences where I have navigated these truths and found my way back to the center again. You can apply these experiences and these teachings to your own life and liberate yourself from living in the constructs we have created for ourselves on this planet at this time.

Living in human form is supposed to be expansive because, by living in a body, we have the ability to touch, feel, and hold each other. Earthly life allows for experiences you cannot have in a Spirit form. My hope is that we can take the expansion of both worlds—physical and non-physical—to understand the gift of experiencing our world in a human body. We can learn to use our human body and our body's vast wisdom to generate higher vibrations and more love rather than constantly living by rules that create more fear. My truth and your truth are one and the same. And when we can co-create and collaborate with each other and with Spirit, we have the ability to make this beautiful Mother Earth, *our* beautiful Mother Earth, thrive again. I *know* we can walk ourselves through this climate crisis that *we* as a society have created and regenerate the earth in the most profound way.

I was reading an article about *the great bloom* that is taking place in California after some of the devastating wildfires decimated everything in their paths. And what is coming forward after this devastation are acres of beautiful wildflowers. Such rich wildflowers that you can actually see them from space! The earth knows how to care for itself when it folds back into its origin. And that is what we are being asked to do. Right now, we are in the middle of a human wildfire. Let's know and have faith that we can regenerate something even more beautiful on the other side of this. Let's stop trying to fix something that isn't broken in the first place. We aren't broken. The earth isn't broken. That is *the big illusion*. It's very human to define and label experiences and try to make sense of or order out of them. We have defined this situation as broken; thus, we must *do* something or *fix* something in order to feel productive. Everybody has their vision of how this looks, and we are continually letting others know they are doing it wrong. We are so profoundly getting in each other's way.

Divine Mother says, "Stop, pause, and listen." The situation we are in is like when our bodies are out of alignment—they give us a big nudge. If we don't hear it, they will give us another one and another one. The earth is doing the same thing. We are out of alignment, and the earth is responding to that. We are a part of this earth, and the earth's wisdom is saying, "I will take care of myself, just as your body will take care of you." The earth asks us to co-create because every living thing is one extraordinary vibration of love. And we have the ability to rise above what is today to the super blooms of tomorrow.

All of the messaging I have received in writing this book is that of hope. There is hope for us as a human race, and there is hope for us on this planet. I often teach that the catalyst for change is often due to living in discomfort. And we are genuinely in discomfort. So let us work together, live together, co-create together—not in fear, but in love—and expand that vibration throughout the world and see what happens. I love you all and am holding the space for this planet to unite, regenerate, rejuvenate, and remember who we are. I hope this book will be a helpful tool on your journey.

We are here to be ministering angels for each other, so go forth to love each other and to serve for the highest and best good of all.

With all my heart, thank you for taking the time to walk this journey with me.

PART I

Our Human Experience

Body Wisdom

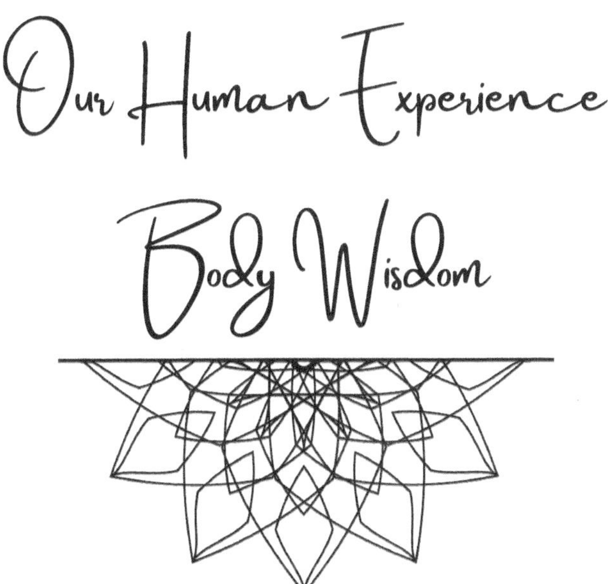

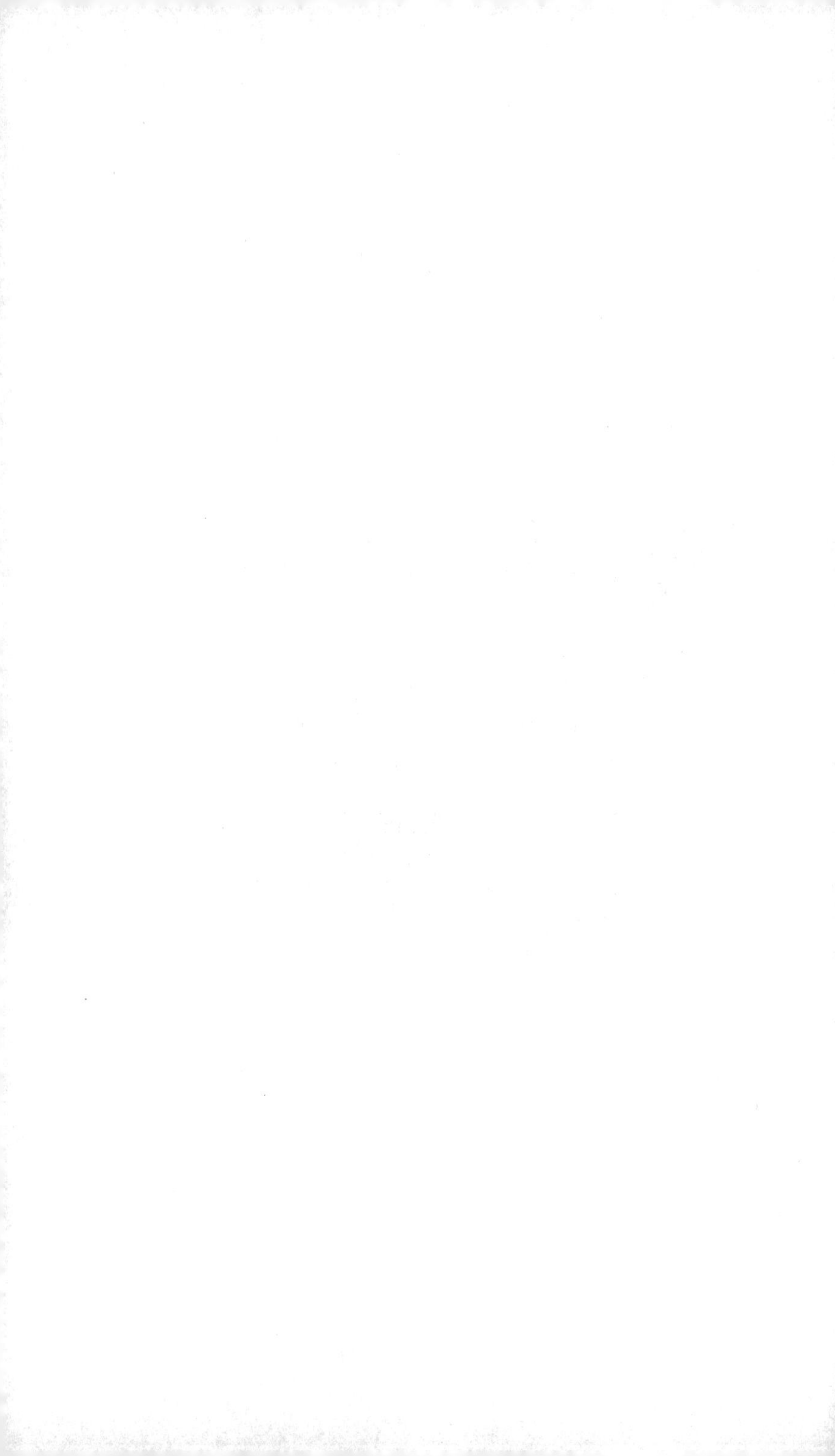

The first three chapters describe challenging experiences I've faced and how I applied my body's wisdom guided by the Sacred Truths to help me navigate each circumstance.

Chapter 1

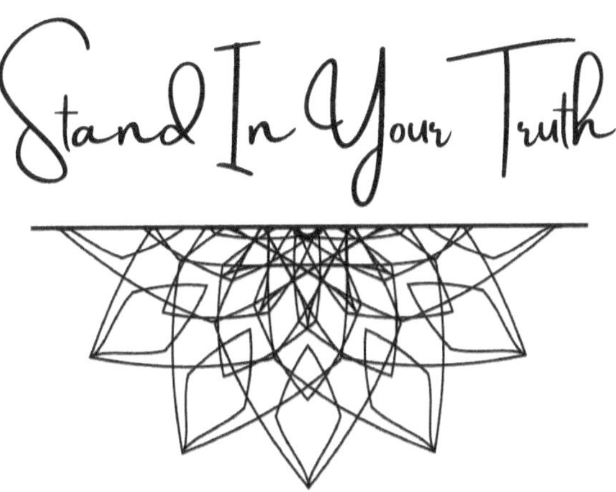

Stand In Your Truth

First Sacred Truth
Divine Manifestation

Our life is spun together like an intricate web, each experience energetically and experientially building upon and influencing future endeavors. A crack in our foundation will eventually reveal itself at some point in our life's journey, at which time we will have a choice: to either address it and begin the healing process or bury it deeper. If the latter, it *will* arise again later, at which time we are faced again with the choice. And again. And again—until we begin healing. Everything from birth forward is dependent upon the foundational love we receive and create within the First Sacred Truth: Divine Manifestation. When we find alignment with this Sacred Truth, we are able to create anything.

The intention of Divine Manifestation is to create an energetic vessel to hold and ground Divine Light and Love in the sacredness of your physical body. Foundationally, all things must be rooted in love to be fully aligned with our truth. Living in Divine Manifestation creates an unbreakable container, one which holds the Light we shine within ourselves and upon others. It is the Light of Spirit. Creating this Spiritual groundwork allows you to manifest and maintain constant, relentless sacredness within your body, home, relationships, community, environment, and for Mother Earth. Living into the truth of Divine Manifestation inspires all potentiality to exist.

The body's energy center correlated with Divine Manifestation is the Muladhara (Moola-dhaa-ruh), or first chakra, and is located at the very base of the spine. When I think about the attributes of this energy center, I consider grounding, foundation, safety, stability, security, family, nurturing, survival, health, and the element of earth. Consider the first chakra as coming home. It's the container holding and supporting all other Truths. As we enter a new beginning into a human body, this is where the union of our physical and Spiritual journey begins.

Just as we receive Divine Messaging from our higher self, our body is also in constant communication in the form of body wisdom. It can show up as a *gut feeling* when something doesn't feel right or "chills" when something exciting happens. Our body's wisdom is aware of every emotional vibration we hold. When the vibration is high, we thrive and find ease. When it is consistently low, we fall into survival mode, eventually resulting in *dis*-ease. I recommend listening when your body expresses in a whisper rather than a roar. Unfortunately, our society is not so great at pausing and being attentive to the subtleties of our body's communication. It requires making a ritual out of taking a respite, going inward, and observing how you are feeling—asking yourself questions and honoring your truest response. We all know how easy it is to pass things off as nothing as we continually get wrapped up in our busy life.

Your body is sacred. It's your greatest asset and communicator. If it doesn't feel right, then something isn't right. Spirit resides within you and will communicate everything you need to know. Open your heart and quiet your mind long enough to receive the response. You deserve to thrive.

My New Beginning

I am a child of adoption. My birth mother found out she was pregnant during her first year in college while home in Minnesota on Christmas break. She was nineteen and unmarried. The only people who knew about the pregnancy were her parents and brother. Pregnant teens in the 1960s had few options. Her parents thought it best for her to return to Colorado, where she had been going to school. She spent the remainder of her pregnancy in a home for unwed mothers.

I entered the world early in the morning of July 25, 1967. My birth mother was only allowed to hold me for one brief moment after I was born before the nurses took me away. The only visitor upon my birth was my paternal grandmother. It would be 25 years before I would embrace or see my birth mother again. She was advised to "Just move on with your life. It's best for you and the baby not to get attached." And just like that, the chord had been cut, both literally and figuratively.

I was placed in foster care while Catholic Charities made arrangements with my new adoptive parents. As the social worker brought me from Denver to Saint Paul, she learned I was the youngest baby to ever fly on that airline. Upon my arrival in Minnesota, I was placed briefly in another foster family's care before meeting my forever family, where I was welcomed with love by my mom, dad, and adopted brother from a different birth mother, Tim.

My parents integrated the understanding that I was adopted from a very young age. I know that because I don't remember getting "the talk" about where I came from or how I landed in their home. I simply always knew I was adopted. As a very young girl, I tried to make sense of how this whole adoption thing worked. Based on my mom and dad telling me they "chose" me, I envisioned that all babies who needed to be adopted were swaddled in bassinets, positioned on giant trays, and placed in a display case—like a donut shop. Each morning, workers would carefully prepare a new batch of babies. Meanwhile, an anxious and anticipatory line of adoptive parents got in a queue outside, waiting to come in and *choose* which baby they wanted. This scenario made me feel special—like I was the donut with frosting and sprinkles—and my parents picked *me*.

Around the age of ten, I asked my mom why they didn't have their own kids, to which she simply said, "We realized we weren't able to have children, so we decided to adopt." True to my mom, her response was very matter-of-fact; no fuss nor drama needed. "As soon as I held you in my arms, it felt like you were mine, and I didn't dwell on how you got there." My mom, Mary, had humble beginnings, growing up as a farm girl in a small town in Iowa. I believe her upbringing is what created such a strong, intelligent, and supportive woman—an ER nurse who led by example.

My mom instilled unwavering confidence in me. I grew up knowing that I could do anything. Her mothering was the ideal combination of nurturing and independence. As an ER nurse, she worked all sorts of crazy hours while also running our household, always the can-do kind of role model. Whenever I complained about something unreasonable, her go-to response was simply "like it or lump it," a phrase that immediately shut my brother and me down—in the best way. To this day, I still believe there isn't anything my mom doesn't know or can't solve. If I can't figure something out or need someone to confide in, I call my mom. The greatest gift she's given me—among many—is a sense of confidence and stability. Without a doubt, I knew she deeply loved me and was there for me no matter what.

My dad and I were also very close. He made sure there wasn't a moment I didn't feel unconditionally loved and wanted. He was the kindest *gentle*man I have ever known. He was also hilarious in an "I-don't-realize-I'm-being-funny" sort of way. After he said something, there was a look of surprise on his face that left everyone laughing yet also wondering, "Is he serious?" My husband is convinced that my dad absolutely knew he was being funny and spent a lifetime of "pulling one over" on all of us.

My dad, by nature, was always concerned about my well-being. He made a habit of circling the house to check in on me. I'd hear him wandering about, yelling my name, "Suzy! Hey Suz? Where you at?" I'd receive daily knocks on my bedroom door, "Hey Suz, you in there?" I'd answer with an, "I'm here. What do you need?" Without fail, his response was, "Oh, okay; just checking."

One morning, I was getting ready for school and was frustrated with how my hair looked. It had gotten all flat from sleeping on it. The day prior, I had gotten my first *real* haircut that was not at the kitchen table with a pair of giant sewing shears. I left the salon with my hair blown out and barrel-rolled, looking just like Toni Tenille. It was *the* haircut of the modern 1970s woman.

That morning, I was determined to fix my lifeless hair. My mom had already left for work, and I had never used a curling iron. I plugged the curling iron in and tried to figure out how to wrap my hair around it without getting burned. My dad came into the bathroom and said he curled his hair all the time and would do it for me. *Hmm*...I thought to myself. This seemed a bit fishy since my dad was bald on top and had the monk ring since he was in his early thirties. I looked him straight in the eyes to decipher the situation. I got his first and only poker face looking back at me. Out of sheer desperation, I took a gamble and let him do it. As he put the first strand of hair around the iron, it was clear I had made the wrong decision.

My parents were thoughtful about ensuring my brother and I never felt weird about being adopted. Every time we'd drive by the Johnsons' house in our neighborhood, my dad would say: "Did you know that Anna and May are adopted?" And every time, I'd simply say, "Yep, Dad, I do know they are adopted." My parents also shared everything they knew about my birth mother—mostly from the standardized form she filled out. The three things that stuck with me were that she was a model, liked swimming, and was petite. I am also very petite. My parents specifically used that word to describe me. I think it sounded sweet, better than short, or strangely small. My mom tells me I weighed 25 pounds when I began kindergarten. "The best things come in small packages," my parents would say over and over again. They did a fantastic job helping me feel special and building my self-esteem. I had a wonderful childhood and felt very, very loved.

As a kid, adoption was not usually on my mind. But occasionally, on my birthday, I would wonder if my birth mom thought of me; I'd get a little curious if she wondered where I was or how I was doing. I later found out after meeting my birth Grandmother that she used to wait outside one of the local elementary schools to see if she could find me in the sea of kids running to their buses.

I do remember having a strong desire for someone to look like me. In 5th grade, I had a friend with similarly colored hair, freckles, and brown eyes. I always wanted to wear matching clothing with her, so people thought we were sisters or, even better, twins. I only remember one time when a childhood friend said something cruel about being adopted. We were in a fight at the park. She said, "At least my parents wanted me." I ran home and cried, not because I believed what she said but because it surprised me that my best friend could be that mean.

Overall, my adopted life was pretty amazing. It wasn't until I had my first daughter that I began to question and consider how critical those first days and weeks of bonding contributed to building a foundation of feeling safe. I felt that something about her birth experience instigated an unsettled awakening within me. I labored for about 24 hours. After almost three hours of pushing, my daughter finally arrived at 1:10 a.m. The nurses got her washed up, and I attempted to breastfeed her for the first time. I swaddled her, and everyone settled into sleep. My hubby was on a pull-out, and Madeline was in her bassinet beside my hospital bed. I had the option of sending her to the nursery for a couple of hours to get better rest, but that felt out of the question. There was no way she was going to be out of my sight.

All was quiet in the room as Joe and Madeline drifted off. On the other hand, I lay in my bed, curled up in the fetal position, shaking uncontrollably. I went in and out of a surreal conscious and unconscious state. It was almost as if I was reliving a trauma but couldn't identify it. I felt terrified—like I was in shock and completely out of control of my body and emotions. My labor was difficult, but this reaction didn't feel like it came from this birthing experience. Instead, my body's wisdom felt as if it was expressing and releasing something from a different time. Finally, at about 6 a.m., Madeline began to stir. The nurse came in to take my vitals and get me going for the day. The episode had somewhat subsided. I snapped into my role as a new mother and left whatever that episode was behind—or so I thought.

A couple of years later, I was standing in the gift-wrapping aisle at Target. My inner voice said to turn around and look down. As I did, I saw a displaced book on the shelf entitled *Twenty Things Adopted Kids Wish Their Adoptive Parents Knew* by Sherrie Eldridge. When I saw the title, I knew I had to buy it. I dove into it as soon as I got home.

The first chapter was about hidden losses. In this chapter, Sherrie Eldridge writes that an adopted child's earliest experience is the loss of their birth parents. She quotes Dr. David M. Brodzinsky and Dr. Marshall D. Scheckter, a psychologist and a psychiatrist specializing in adoption, from their book, *Being Adopted,* "Loss for the adoptee is unlike the losses we have come to expect in a lifetime, such as death and divorce. Instead, adoption is more pervasive, less socially recognized, and more profound." In his book, *The Spirit Of Open Adoption,* James Gritter explains, "The pain of adoption is not something that happens to a person; it is the person. It is virtually impossible to describe because the pain is so primal."

I may not have a visual reference for this experience, but I can guarantee that an intangible, somatic memory is stored in my body relating to abandonment and loss. Renowned child psychoanalyst Selma Fraiberg writes: "What is remembered or preserved is anxiety, a primitive kind of terror, which returns in waves later in life. Loss and danger of loss of love become recurrent themes or life patterns."

I sometimes reflect on those first few weeks of life. I wonder how I must have felt each time I transitioned to a new foster home with new people, sounds, and smells before I landed in my forever home. When I read this following passage, it unearthed a massive wound. Something that I stored so deeply inside me began to come out. The chapter was entitled "Entering Your Child's World."

Adoption day finally arrives, the day that at times seemed an eternity away. The home studies are over. The "what ifs" are behind you…as you carry the baby into her new home for everyone to see. "Isn't she beautiful!" they all say one after another. Grandparents hold her first, then the aunts and uncles. The baby lies quietly in each person's arms, seemingly oblivious to all that is happening around her. However, no one knows that beneath that crisp white dress is a tiny grieving heart…a heart that wonders where my mom is? Her smell. The sound of her voice. Her heartbeat. Her body. Where did she go? Such is the primal loss that your adopted baby experiences on the day she comes home.

After reading that passage, I remember sitting in the bathtub and bursting into tears. This book validated emotions, beliefs, and behaviors I had carried and exhibited throughout my entire life but couldn't put into words or understand. At that moment, I had an experience as if I was giving witness to myself as an infant, trying to feel safe. I felt compassion and grief for this tiny baby who was me. At the same time, I felt guilty for having these instinctual emotions. I do not want to hurt my parents' feelings because they did *everything* right. They loved and nurtured me so beautifully. They supported me in every way. There is absolutely nothing that I could have asked for that would have made my experience growing up more perfect. It was an idyllic childhood with idyllic parents. To this day, I feel like it was a miracle that I landed in this family because it is just so special, and I have always felt immensely loved. I am also so grateful to my birth mother. She loved me while I was in utero and wanted the best for me. She made an incredible sacrifice by giving me life and also by giving me away. I know this wasn't easy for her or her family. All of the intentions and love that I received were beautiful.

That book was a gift to me. I discovered my foundation had a big crack that needed my attention and love. Something very primal within me doesn't yet *know* I am safe without all of my loved ones surrounding me. For me, this translates into an inability to trust the permanence of relationships. I don't feel that my immediate family is going to walk away from me. I fear that they will be taken away from me by something out of their control, like death. My biggest fear is losing them and being abandoned. This fear became far more pronounced after my episode in the hospital following the birth of my first daughter. When loved ones leave, as in going to school, work, or on a trip, I don't trust I will see them again. And the truth is that I may not. But how I experience each parting seems different than what most people feel.

I have a family dog named Winnie. She's an Australian shepherd. When my kids were little, Winnie would literally herd them when they were running in the yard. She'd nip at their heels, desperately trying to gather them together. *That is how I feel.* I have constant underlying anxiety, needing to know that my kids (now grown adults) are safe. I am stuffing a persistent undercurrent of fear and am exhibiting the same instinctual behavior as my dog, Winnie. It is rooted that deep within me. Winnifred also likes to sit in the window and keep watch on the house. She barks at everything—even when the wind blows. One day—truly, most days—Winnie was howling at nothing. As I went over to calm her down, I said, "Winnie, you are imagining threats that are not there." I thought to myself, *Hmmm, that feels familiar.*

Until I began this quest for healing, I never understood why I had such difficulty saying goodbye to loved ones. I came to discover that my way of managing this anxiety was by being absolutely vigilant about saying, "I love you," when we parted ways. To this day, I text this to my girls and my mom every night before bed. It helps me know I have done all I can. I couldn't express this as an infant before being separated from my birth mom. I didn't have a voice. And now I do. So, should anything happen to my sacred people or me, it helps me to know that the words "I love you" were the last ones they heard.

The Gift

The common thread that sews our human experiences together is the foundational need for safety, security, and stability. In order to thrive, we must know we are physically and emotionally safe. So how do we heal from foundational issues and find our way back into our Truth and Divine Manifestation? We all want to live in the abundance of manifestation rather than scarcity and survival. The answer lies in attuning to our sacred vessel, the human body. Take the time to pause and listen to its beautiful language, your body's wisdom. It is Spirit speaking through physical experiences.

Mine expressed itself years ago after the birth of my first daughter. My body said it was time to begin unraveling the pain of abandonment. Unfortunately, I believe people subscribe to the misnomer that there is a time limit for how long the healing process should take. We come into a body to explore, learn, expand, and grow. This wound of abandonment is a part of my life's journey. Every step I take forward awakens a new gift within me, and I firmly believe that with every challenge comes a remarkable reward. So often, it is intangible. By listening to my body's wisdom, I can understand it in an incredibly intimate way.

The most profound gift that I have received from growing up in such a fantastic home is understanding how to love fearlessly. Of course, it doesn't mean that I am not afraid. But it does mean that even though I struggle with the fear of losing the people I love, I step into my relationships with a fully open heart despite it all. Because I put trust in my higher self, Spirit, and the intangible to guide me through, I divinely manifested my hubby and three daughters—or as we call ourselves, "The Fab Five."

Help In Healing Through Divine Manifestation

After hearing a bit about my journey, I hope you can take the time to dig into your own experiences. Notice if there is a need to examine some things in your life and heal your foundation. In addition to the yoga and meditation practices that I'm providing, I have some thoughtful questions for you to take into your meditation time as well as helpful suggestions to get yourself grounded in your beautiful body and to feel nurtured by the Spirit of Mother Earth.

• Sit still and listen! Carve out time each day to just be alone with yourself and Spirit. Tune into the wisdom that comes forward. Everyone receives this insight differently, so be patient with yourself and see how your inner voice shares its story.

• Shift your perspective as you observe your experiences. Be a witness rather than a participant to discern these experiences in your life objectively.

• Give and receive the gift of touch (massage, hands-on healing, hugs).

• Connect intimately with the earth by taking nature walks or standing barefoot in the grass. Use your senses to take in the beauty of your surroundings.

• Nature provides us with the vibration of unconditional love. Find some stillness on your walk and take in the earth's vibration. Surrender what isn't serving you and just receive. Notice how your body is responding.

• Get your hands in the dirt, try gardening, and eat root vegetables.

• Do the recorded Grounding Meditation I am offering each morning and evening. Be present with your body and feel your connection to the earth. Notice your stress levels throughout the day. Notice your quality of sleep by incorporating these before bed.

Divine Manifestation Affirmation

"I am the Light of Divine Manifestation. Through this Sacred Truth, I have a knowingness that I am safe and deeply grounded to Mother Earth. I am a sacred vessel, cradling and nurturing my Soul Light of Divinity within me."

Journal Questions

As you ponder each question, ask yourself, "Am I being honest with myself?" This can be a lovely conversation between yourself and Spirit. Spirit knows all the answers and is compassionate and patient as you find the courage to face the truth in your answers.

• Does your foundation have any cracks (past and present) that need your attention?

• Do you feel grounded, stable, and safe?

• Are you meeting your foundational needs? If not, what are actionable steps you can take to make this happen?

• Do you feel loved by yourself and others?

• Do you accept love from yourself and others?

• Is there wounding that requires your attention?

• Are you able to describe or put a name to your wounding?

• Do you need help exploring this wounding?

As you embark on your healing journey, begin by sending up a prayer to your beautiful Spirit Guides. They are just waiting to step in to support you. But it must be at your request. They will never override your freedom of choice. You can also reach out for support from a trusted friend, family member, mental healthcare provider, or me. You are never alone.

Yoga & Meditation

My channeled yoga class guides you through long, stabilizing postures in which you begin to feel your connection and support from the earth. The meditation mirrors the yoga class. I encourage long, steady breathing and feeling the earth's resonant embrace. To access your classes, scan the QR code or visit the link.

https://bit.ly/3W3sueX

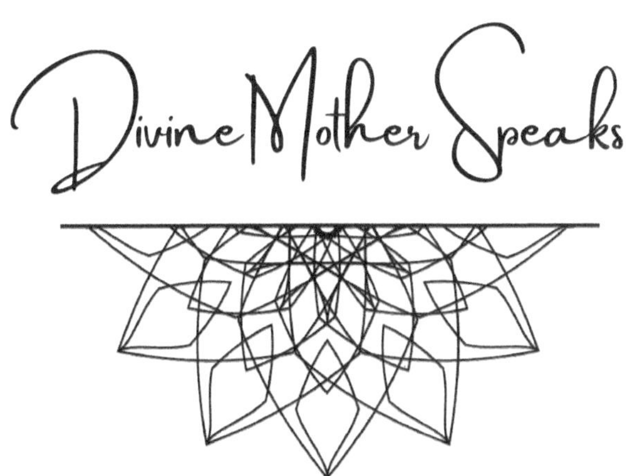

Divine Manifestation

Beloved Ones,

Visualize a container made of diamonds. And what is held within this container is diamond white light. This container and its contents are absolute perfection and give off the most magnificent reflection of a full spectrum of light—a rainbow ray. This container is your human body. What is held within is your soul and an unbreakable, everlasting bond with Spirit.

You are the perfect vessel for Spirit to reside within. You embody the perfection of Spirit. What creates your perfection is love. Love is Spirit, and Spirit is love. And love is the essence and the foundation of who you are. Love is infinite abundance and pure manifestation. When you remember this truth, you have created the grounded stability for everything else in your life to so brilliantly build upon. When you live in alignment with this truth, you have the ability to create miracles.

With Loving Kindness,

Divine Mother

Chapter 2

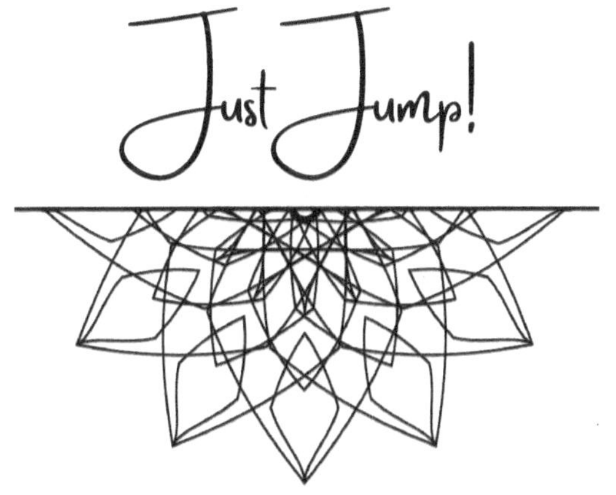

Second Sacred Truth
Divine Rebirth

"Divine Rebirth means that every day, out of love for yourself, out of love for the sacredness of who you are, you must tend to the Divinity and that of the blessed life force that is continually generating within you." –BT

Imagine standing with each of your feet planted on opposite banks of a calm, easy-flowing river. The river represents the flow of your Divine life and one of endless spectacular opportunities, carrying you gently and effortlessly when you allow it. When we experience indecisiveness, it's as if each foot digs in deeper on either side of the river—fearful and resistant to change. The imagery of not trusting ourselves—not taking the leap of faith and letting our life river flow—is the clairvoyant image I often receive when guiding a client who is navigating anxiety about change. The fear of the unknown paralyzes them from taking a leap of faith. Change is inevitable and a natural part of life. Resistance to this change is like putting your feet down in the middle of the river, attempting to stop the flow. That takes immense effort and is not sustainable. The message I am offering is to trust your Divine Inner Wisdom and the natural flow of life and just jump! Allow the divinity of your river to carry you!

The Second Sacred Truth is Divine Rebirth and is associated with our second chakra, Svadhisthana (Sva-dee-stah-nuh). For women, it aligns within our womb, the source of creation, and is the seat of passion and change.

The element of the second chakra is water which conjures movement, flow, purification, and renewal. It supports personal expansion and the formation of identity through relationships with others and the world.

Divine Rebirth is about evolving and shape-shifting in and out of our comfort zone. It's taking what we understand of the first chakra, Divine Manifestation, as a place to anchor our Divine Light and putting that into movement and flow by regenerating this Light or life force into a soul rebirth. In other words, we have established our stable foundation, filled with pure diamond white Light; now let's create! Whether it's personal transformation and enlightenment within, discovering your life's purpose, or manifesting better health, a new relationship, career, or home, let's explore Divine Rebirth, plant the seeds of change, and give birth to something new.

I often ask my students and clients to remember a time in their lives when they felt most passionate and unlimited in their potential. Whether encountering a powerful experience in the present or visualizing it from the past, we can tap into this fierce vibration, aligning us with manifestation. In this chapter, I share two very different experiences in my life: one, the powerful memory of playing "king of the mountain" as a child with my brother and his friends on warm summer evenings in Minnesota, and second, memories of many years of being bullied as a teen. Each, in turn, affected my self-worth and how I moved through the world in drastically different ways.

King of the Mountain

When I was a little girl, one of my favorite things to do was run around outside in the summertime, barefoot, with as little clothing on as possible so that I could feel the warm, humid air on my skin and the earth under my feet. I grew up in a sweet little suburb of St. Paul, Minnesota. We had a bunch of kids who lived on our block, or what I called "the island." The island was comprised of about 12 homes that were connected by our backyards, six on each side, with no fences and no streets intersecting the island. This gave us kids lots of running and hiding space to go out in the evenings, after dinner, and "get a game going." My brother and I were generally the organizers of our games, making multiple phone calls to see who could come out and play. We would make lists of available friends, which then determined what game we'd entertain ourselves with that night. Sometimes it was ditch, kick the can or four square. If we had enough kids, we'd play capture the flag or touch football. Because our house had the biggest and flattest backyard, it became the prime meeting location for our games.

I most enjoyed running around with my older brother and his friends because I was extremely competitive, and the boys always provided a significant challenge. I just loved to run, tumble, and move my body. One of my favorite games was "king of the mountain." Our next-door neighbor had a good-sized hill, so all of us kids would run to the top and try to push each other down the "mountain." The last one standing became king—or queen, in my case. I certainly was not the strongest kid, but I always felt agile and difficult to catch. Running with the boys made me feel powerful because no one babied me. And the laughter as we'd hurl ourselves at each other while tumbling down the hill is one of my favorite childhood memories.

I share this story with you because when I think about that time, it makes me smile and reminds me of feeling uninhibited joy and freedom. I think about how magical the summer nights were growing up in the Midwest— running barefoot and the smell of the grass and cottonwood trees. I think about how we would giggle and strategize about the best hiding spot. My focus was not on what I looked like or the clothing I wore. I didn't care that I was small. In fact, it made me proud because it never stopped me from participating in anything. I had an I'll-show-you-what-I'm-made-of kind of attitude. Moving my body makes me feel powerful-even to this day. This was a time in my life when I loved *into* the gifts that I was given as a spirited, free-flowing, athletic kid, and they served me well.

Then Came Junior High

It was the fall of seventh grade and my first year in junior high. My junior high melded together about six elementary schools, so it felt really big. Leading up to the school year, I remember my mom telling me about all of the extra-curricular activities that were offered. I loved to swim, so I joined the swim team. Our swim team had a great coach and an amazing reputation. We were undefeated, winning first in state all three years I was on the team. Regardless of one's ability, our coach made everyone feel like a contributing part of the team. The bus rides to and from the swim meets were also super inclusive—everyone was singing and laughing. As we approached our opposing school, we'd open the windows on the bus and chant our school song as loud as we could so everyone knew we were coming. Because we won every meet, it was even more fun to do the same thing on our return to school.

I also loved to sing and signed up for choir. Girls choir met first thing in the morning during homeroom and was filled with seventh through ninth-graders. We were about a month into the school year, and I was sitting in my chair, waiting for the choir director to come in and begin. Suddenly, an eighth-grader named Dana abruptly grabbed me by my shirt and dragged me out of class. I was pulled around the corner and shoved into the wall. For the first time in my life, I wished I was bigger. Not even close to five feet tall and probably 80 pounds soaking wet, I was surrounded by a sea of eighth and ninth-grade boys and girls. The ninth graders looked like adults to me. As I was processing what was happening, I could feel my face flush and my heart beating out of my chest. I was actually worried that I might wet my pants because I was so scared.

I had no idea what was happening; honestly, I am not certain most of the kids around me knew either. They said some aggressive and threatening things and then just let me go back into class. Trying not to cry, I made my way back to my seat. No one, including my very kind choir teacher, knew what had just occurred. I said nothing, terrified it would happen again if I told anyone.

As the year progressed, I remember being so excited about a choir sleepover at my school. We brought sleeping bags, roller skates, food, and music. It should have been a really fun event. I tried to keep to a corner of the school that was away from Dana and her pack of friends. As I was sitting by the wall, taking a break from roller skating, Dana and her crew came by. She began yelling at me, then picked up my pillow and hit me repeatedly with it, slamming my head against the concrete wall. Everybody just stood by and watched. No one interceded or threw me a lifeline. As I reflect on that experience, I wonder—*Where was that feisty, run-around-with-the-boys, king-of-the-mountain girl?* She was frozen in shame and fear, allowing Dana to continue the humiliation. I felt that taking any action would only make it worse.

Dana was my best friend's cousin. Let's just say my best friend was not helpful in alleviating the bullying throughout the school year. The name-calling, threats, and shoves went on for several months. Then, out of the blue, Dana sat down beside me in choir and apologized. I just looked at her with a blank stare, not sure how to react. I felt certain she was lying, trying another way to degrade me. My response was a simple, non-emotional, and somewhat surprised, "Okay?" In hindsight, I believe she was looking for some sort of appreciation for her gesture. Unfortunately, my reaction, or lack thereof, made her angry. So she called me a bitch and stormed away.

Eventually, Dana grew tired of me and my non-reaction and moved on. The abuse finally subsided that spring. But, in the summer leading up to eighth grade, a new group led by my three closest friends decided they would pick up where Dana left off. The torment spread like a cancer. Soon no one wanted to be associated with me, worried they, too, would receive the wrath of the most popular kids in my grade.

Once school began, I would be surprised each day that yet another friend or even someone I didn't know would show up with a nasty note or harassing word. At my school, there were three choice words these girls would use to disrespect one another. They were bitch, whore, or wench. Super creative, right? They could be used singularly, interchangeably, or…if they were really feeling astute with their words, *a trifecta*. So the end of my school day would look something like this. I'd be waiting for my bus, and any number of girls would approach me. They'd say how sorry they were for their behavior and hand me their well-crafted "apology" note. I ended up with a drawer full of "apology" notes reminding me—in the event I forgot— that I was a whore, bitch, wench, or potentially the whole trifecta, depending on their mood. Sometimes I imagined them sitting in class, really immersing themselves in their writing skills, thinking, "Hmm. What to say? What. To. Say. Oh, I know, I'll call her a …" So clever.

There were other days in which the bullying was more physical. I was pulled into the showers after gym class, cornered in the bathroom, then slammed against the wall, and sometimes threatened to be locked in a locker. However, this particular experience was the pinnacle of humiliation and truly messed with my heart and my trust.

Ever since the beginning of seventh grade, I had a mad crush on this boy in my class. He happened to be very good friends with the lead bully. One Friday night, he was having a party. That evening, out of the blue, he called me and asked if I wanted to come over. He sounded kind and sincere—like it was an oversight that I wasn't invited. He went on to say how sorry he was for the way I had been treated. Naively, I was taken in by his charm and said, "Really? I'll have to ask my parents if I can get a ride." A moment later, several kids who had been listening in from another phone began laughing hysterically at me. They dropped the trifecta, adding how stupid I was, then hung up. I remember sitting in my room that night, looking out the window above my bed, thinking, if I died tonight, maybe someone might actually feel bad and consider the damage caused by how they behaved. I don't believe I was ever suicidal; I just fantasized about what it would feel like to have someone—anyone—genuinely care and apologize.

The awful words that were spoken to me were definitely the harshest and most damaging part of my experience. A shove only lasted a second, but the words began to take root inside of me. I tried to make light of it, but I knew I was losing trust in everyone. There was a time when I didn't feel I had a single friend. For an entire semester, I ate my lunch by my locker because I was afraid to go down to the lunchroom and sit alone or, worse yet, have someone say they didn't want me to sit there and have to move. At that time, I didn't feel like I had a shred of dignity or self-worth left. I was in full-on survival. And then I met Lynn.

The Gift of a Lifetime

I remember seeing Lynn for the first time in seventh grade at the roller rink. She was skating with her brother-in-law, who I mistook to be her boyfriend. It was 1980, and Lynn had this amazing mane of wild blonde hair and wore large aviator-style glasses. She looked as if she was 20 years old, which I thought was so cool. It was two years later before we were introduced—the summer leading into ninth grade. From the moment I met her, I thought she was the absolute funniest person alive. Lynn and I immediately understood that we had the ability to make each other laugh in a way no one else could. To this day, she's the one person I should not sit by at a serious event.

That summer, we spent many nights sleeping out on her sun porch. It was my mission to make her laugh so hard that either iced tea would come out her nose or she'd wet her pants. When she stayed at my house, she would find some sort of costume to put on while I was in the bathroom getting ready for bed. My favorite ensemble was my brother's second-grade horned-rimmed glasses from the 70s, a button-down shirt, and a bowtie. It wasn't so much about what she was wearing, but how she could contort her face in the strangest way. I absolutely could not control my laughter. After relentlessly pleading with my parents to allow our sleepovers, each time, we inevitably awoke my poor sleeping mom, who had to be up at 4 a.m. for work.

One thing that I love about Lynnie is that absolutely nothing embarrasses her. At any given moment, no matter the location, she might break into a full-on Carol Burnett Tarzan call or one of her perfected impressions. I remember one night, we met this guy named Ewan. She talked to him for a while and got his phone number. Later that night, Lynn decided to call him using her spot-on Scottish accent—think Ewan McGregor. There was no answer, so she left this message, "Ewan! I've got the clap. You've got to get yourself checked!" and then hung up. The last time I went to visit Lynn in Seattle, she had a set of "Billy Bob" teeth that she keeps in the glove box of her car. Simply to amuse herself, when she's stuck in Seattle traffic—which is often—she pops them in and smiles at the car next to her. She makes certain to hold her gaze long enough that they lock eyes.

The gift and rebirth that Lynn offered me was unconditional love and the ability to trust in someone again. The way Lynn lives her life is with pure freedom of expression and an unabashed outpouring of joy and laughter. Lynn speaks her truth in a way that I had never experienced before, and she is true to that today. Before we met, she heard all of the gossip about me and was warned not to be my friend. None of it mattered because she was going to find out for herself. She expanded my view of the world and showed me what it looks like to love myself no matter what anyone else thinks about me or does to me.

Over the years, our lives have ebbed and flowed, but she has remained my very best friend and soul sister from the day we met. We were each other's maid of honor and now have a gaggle of grown daughters. Our gatherings are bigger than life. Lynnie was and forever will be one of the greatest gifts given to me. She came into my life when I so desperately needed a friend. She *saw* me—I mean really saw me—heart and soul. I will forever be grateful for our friendship.

This is a poem that Lynn recently sent me. I feel that she has always lived her life as if her bowl was near empty—

never, ever taking a moment for granted. I love you so
much, my sweet friend.

I counted my years
and realized that
I have less time to live by,
than I have lived so far.
I have more past than future.
I feel like that girl who got a bowl of cherries.
At first, she gobbled them,
but when she realized there were only few left,
she began to taste them intensely.
I no longer have time to deal with mediocrity.
I do not want to be in meetings where flamed egos parade.
I am bothered by the envious,
who seek to discredit the most able,
to usurp their places, coveting their seats,
talent, achievements and luck.
I do not have time for endless conversations,
useless to discuss about the lives of others
who are not part of mine.
I no longer have the time to manage
sensitivities of people who, despite their chronological
age, are immature.
I hate to confront those that struggle for power,
those that 'do not debate content, just the labels.'
My time has become scarce to debate labels,
I want the essence.
My soul is in a hurry ...
Not many cherries in my bowl,

I want to live close to human people, very human,
who laugh of their own stumbles,
and away from those turned smug
and overconfident with their triumphs,
away from those filled with self-importance.
The essential is what makes life worthwhile.
And for me, the essentials are enough!
Yes, I'm in a hurry.
I'm in a hurry to live with the intensity that only maturity
can give.
I do not intend to waste any of the remaining cherries.
I am sure they will be exquisite, much more than those
eaten so far.
My goal is to reach the end satisfied
and at peace with my loved ones and my conscience.
And per Confucius "We have two lives
and the second begins when you realize you only have
one."

Poem: Mário de Andrade - The Valuable Time of Maturity

The Gift In Rebirth

The experience of being bullied has been difficult to write about because there are so many emotions packed away, both good and bad. As I sit with my memories, I recognize that some of these emotions are still unresolved, and I struggle to figure out why. In my other chapters, I write about experiences that I had in communion with others.

Even though they were difficult, we co-created something beautiful out of something challenging. In this experience, I was not traveling through the experience in union with these people but in contrast. When you think of the imagery of the river, in those years prior to the bullying, I was just floating along, minding my own business, and enjoying the ride. Then suddenly, I became entangled with these classmates. No matter what I did, I felt anchored to the bottom of the river, continually being pulled under by the current of their abuse. However, no matter how exhausted and disheartened I became, I didn't allow them to drown me in their issues.

It's interesting because when I think about that time in my life, it's as if that teen girl and my adult self are two separate people. Some may describe this as resiliency because I am able to separate the two experiences and move on in my life. However, I look at resiliency as being masterful at compartmentalizing uncomfortable or traumatic experiences for the sake of survival. If we truly want to thrive in this lifetime, we must go within, let those experiences surface, and begin the healing process. This means finding true forgiveness for ourselves and others.

As I observe my teenage self, I feel sad for that kid, but I don't pity her, nor do I want that for her. Pity is one of the lowest vibrations because it is a complete departure from hope. It is a belief that disempowers a person, essentially stating, "I am helpless to resolve my situation and lack the ability to create change for myself—so much so that someone else must do it for me."

When you pity someone else, you are projecting your lack of confidence in them, which ultimately becomes demoralizing. It's forgetting that this person's soul is infinite and can transform whatever experience they are having into a rebirth of something extraordinary. The best way to support someone is by showing compassion rather than pity and, only if requested, assisting in the situation without feeling the need to control it. Inquire about their needs rather than impose an opinion. Then step back and allow them their time of growth, knowing that they are a fully capable human being experiencing a remarkable time of personal transformation.

Bullying so often happens during formative years. Regardless of whether you're a child or an adult, the things people say become beliefs if you allow them in. As I am unpacking this and processing what happened, there are parts that definitely feel incomplete. I've gone into my heart to explore what I need, and the answer is that I really don't know. I do know there is a continuing story from my adoption about abandonment and self-worth—thinking if I were good enough, people wouldn't walk away from me. This experience fed into my hesitation to trust people and the permanency of relationships. I got a really good view of the underbelly of human behavior when faced with the fear of being ostracized from a group.

What I'm also feeling is the wounding from an abrupt loss of innocence. I guess it feels like grief. I'm grieving that child who could run freely, playing king of the mountain, and feeling invincible. Even though I know she's still there, her powerful self can often get buried under beliefs about self-worth. It's possible that I need to dig deeper into my heart and offer compassion to myself and those who treated me poorly. I may never know why they did what they did. And it is doubtful I ever will. What I do know is that someone who behaves badly is not sitting in their truth and couldn't possibly feel very good inside. In the words of Ted Lasso, "Hurt people hurt people." For that, I offer compassion, grace, and forgiveness. That is my road to freedom.

The Gift of Just Jumping!

Do you ever feel like you are being prepared for something greater than you can even imagine? You aren't sure what it is, but there is just a *feeling* you have inside that something really extraordinary is coming. Something so great is just around the corner. You cannot see it, touch it, or understand it because it is inaccessible at the current moment. All you know is that many doors are closing for you. The frustration is mounting because nothing seems to be working in your favor. And...also...there is this indescribable glimmer of hope that resides deep within your heart. It's an inner knowingness that life is going to change in the most profound way, and there is nothing you can do about it but wait with positive intentions and allow it to happen.

In 2020, shortly after Covid hit the U.S., I had the option or opportunity, depending on how you look at it, to walk away from my successful yoga studio, Pure Yoga, that I had built up for over a decade and step into the unknown. My studio had a wonderful reputation, being awarded "Best Yoga Studio" in the river valley for an entire decade. I had top-notch, nurturing, educated instructors and a truly beautiful community of clients.

Prior to this worldwide event, I had very seriously considered selling my studio because it was time to challenge myself and expand on my true passions. I wanted to spend more time with my clients and grow more deeply in my healing ministry. I wanted to release the burden of managing schedules, staffing, and all of the things that go along with a brick & mortar business. I wanted to be with my people and to feel the freedom of being fluid with my time and attention.

In my teachings, I often discuss living in one's dharma. Dharma means to live in and fulfill your life's higher purpose. It's that one thing that excites you when you daydream about it. It gives you a sense of deep satisfaction that this is what you came into this lifetime to do to make this world a better place. My dharma began by leaving a career as a fashion stylist in the film industry and opening Pure Yoga. My desire was to create a place for the community to come together and be nurtured. A place for them to feel safe, let down their daily burdens, heal, and explore their own life, hoping to discover and grow into their true dharma.

I learned so much about myself from this experience and also knew from a place deep inside of me that it was time to find my next lily pad and jump. I put the studio on the market and had a couple of potential buyers. Because of the financial instability due to the pandemic, their financing fell through. My lease was set to renew on June 1st, and due to the pandemic, we were not seeing clients in person yet. On May 30th, I decided regardless if I had a buyer or not, now was the time to leap. I called in the cavalry to help me pack up the studio, and two days later, I began the new adventure that I intuitively felt coming for some time.

It. Was. Liberating. I never once regretted my decision. However, as the weeks and months went on, I began to notice all of the attachments I had to the studio and how I identified myself during that time, which is directly in contrast with the word I just used—liberating. What I know is that attachments keep you stuck in the past and create a sense of frustration, fear, and ambiguity about the future. I was a successful female business owner with a beautiful following of both yoga and healing clients. It was enormously fulfilling, and I strongly identified with these roles.

As the pandemic pushed on and the isolation continued, I lost some of those connections. I busied myself by recreating my offerings and my brand. I found myself going deeper and deeper into silence and pause. During this pause, I recognized how much I relied upon others to feed me and fuel my perception of who I thought I was versus who I truly am. I have experienced some very lonely times for the past couple of years and have also been fairly hard on myself as I am making my way. I'd like to say making my way forward, but it certainly hasn't felt like I'm going forward, backward, or sideways. I am simply here in this space of *now*. My sweet ego is constantly, *constantly* chiming in, reminding me that in this time of silence, people will forget me, that I am becoming irrelevant, and that I'll lose everything that I spent years building. Geesh, who's bullying who now?

The image that comes to me is that I am spiraling deeper and deeper into a spider's web. The more I struggle, the more tangled I become until I feel there is no way out. No hope. No path. I cannot see beyond this sticky web that I chose. I chose to walk away from my business. I chose to walk deeper into this silence and into this pause. It has been so incredibly uncomfortable as I deconstruct old patterns and thoughts of who I am and how I have identified myself for so many years.

Rather than reach out to others, I have chosen to continue to stay in this space of isolation because I KNOW that I am in a time of labor and rebirth. I now have a single-pointed focus and clear determination. I am remembering WHO I AM and why I am on this planet during this time of deep unrest. And when I am able to shed a layer of my ego—release another piece of the facade—I also have had some truly intense and euphoric moments in which I see my beautiful and perfect divinity reflected back at me.

I visualize this image of myself holding my hands open in the wind while watching all that I thought about myself and who I thought I was slowly dissipating into the air until there was nothing left. All of my clients, my ego around titles and accomplishments, my memories of childhood and being bullied as a teen slowly released from my grasp until I am alone, with nothing but me, my Spirit, and my connection to the Divine. I have moments when I see Spirit in everyone and everything, most especially within myself. I am filled up in a way that is completely indescribable. I am brought to tears, to this sense of overwhelm, because I remember that I am a part of the whole. I am forever a ministering angel upon this planet. I feel myself vibrate with joy. And today, as I sit writing this chapter, I feel as if I am doing the greatest work of my life.

Help In Healing Through Divine Rebirth

I chose to share these stories because we all have wounding packed away that our body's wisdom is well aware of. All of these experiences that I share are still a part of my story in this lifetime. And yet, I fervently believe they do not have to define me. I get to choose which powerful experiences I want to take along on my journey. I also get to clear the clutter and release those that no longer serve me. You, too, have this choice. All of these experiences put a fierceness and a fearlessness in me. I'm reminded of that saying, "What doesn't kill you makes you stronger." That twelve-year-old junior-high girl is me. But so is the girl who loved to roll around outside with her brother, playing king of the mountain. And that is what makes me able to step into the unknown over and over. Because I know what it feels like to be powerful and free. I also know what it feels like to have to stand alone in fear. I know what it feels like to have my identity stripped away and rebirth myself—each time expanding the womb to make space for who I am in this moment.

Our "identity" is the ego telling us who we are, based on how we feel at that moment. It isn't real, nor is it accurate. Just like my vision of the river bank, I have a choice. We all have a choice. I often ask myself, "Do I want to stand with my feet so deeply rooted in fear that I cannot evolve into who I came into this lifetime to be?" Because doing nothing and becoming stagnant is a choice. Or—I can dig deeper, find that powerful person I know has always been there, step into the unknown, and just jump!

Earlier in this chapter, I referred to "jumping to a new lily pad." This is the imagery I receive in a healing session when my client desires change, and it feels too daunting. The imagery that shows up is a frog sitting on a lily pad. I am not asking my clients to leap all the way across the pond. I am encouraging them to move forward, taking a small leap to the next lily pad. Then, allow time to pause and assess where they landed. Feel into the situation before they take the next leap.

Divine Rebirth and the second chakra are instrumental in developing flexibility, creativity, and change. If you are in a similar situation, below are some suggestions supporting your journey.

- Simplify your life in a way that allows you to be more fluid and available to opportunities as they show up.
- Recognize and release excessive emotional attachments to *things, people,* and *titles* that are rooted in ego or fear that lower your vibration rather than allow you to feel joyful.
- Free yourself from financial burdens (i.e., downsize your living situation to release financial stress and allow room for flexibility in employment opportunities).
- Do an inventory of *wants* vs. *needs.*
- Invest in experiences vs. material possessions. (The Gen Z population is so great at this!)
- Reach out for help in clearing limiting beliefs.
- Is a lack of control holding you back from change?

- Are you challenged with making a decision? Remember, no decision is also a choice.
- Also, remember that there are no bad decisions. No matter what path you take, there is always something profound to learn from the journey.
- Are you feeling anxious about creating change? Explore what is the root of your fear.
- Are you having issues with co-dependency? Is it difficult for you to do things on your own or trust your decision-making?

Divine Rebirth Affirmation

"I am the Light of Divine Rebirth. Through this Sacred Truth, I have the potential to transform, regenerate, renew, and reawaken all things."

Journal Questions

- Remember a time in your life when you felt the most powerful—with absolute freedom. There may be a few times that come to mind. Journal about how this felt. Find a picture/s that reminds you of this powerful time and put it in a place where you will see it daily.
- If you are daydreaming about a powerful moment from the past, remember that person is still inside of you, fully capable of recreating anything you desire, just as you did during that time in your life.

- Take time to daydream about what you most desire. Allow your thoughts to flow and see where it takes you. Journal about these thoughts.
- REMEMBER…your vibration attunes to how you are feeling in the moment, whether it be remembering a past event or experiencing it in real-time.
- Take advantage of your daydreaming time. The time to set intentions and ask Spirit for help in manifesting these intentions is when your vibration is high and full of life.
- A high-vibrating thought or emotion matches all other high vibrations. That is how manifestation and the Law of Attraction work. (For more about The Law of Attraction, check out *Ask and it is Given*, by Abraham/Hicks).
- While you are daydreaming, notice if the ego continues to interrupt with fearful thoughts and limiting beliefs.
- Journal these beliefs and begin a journey into discovering their origins.
- Once you've discovered the origin of your limiting beliefs, journal about how you can release or neutralize these beliefs. Remember, this is just fear coming forward and the ego trying to keep you small and under control.
- Always, always ask for Spirit and your angels to step in to help. They are awaiting your call and ready to jump in to assist you.

Yoga & Meditation

The yoga class accompanying this chapter is built on flowing, creative movement. It will awaken the hips and support the release of old, un-serving beliefs, thus preparing us for a Divine Rebirth. The meditation's theme is deep visualization of one's most powerful moments. To access your classes, scan the QR code or visit the link.

https://bit.ly/3W3sueX

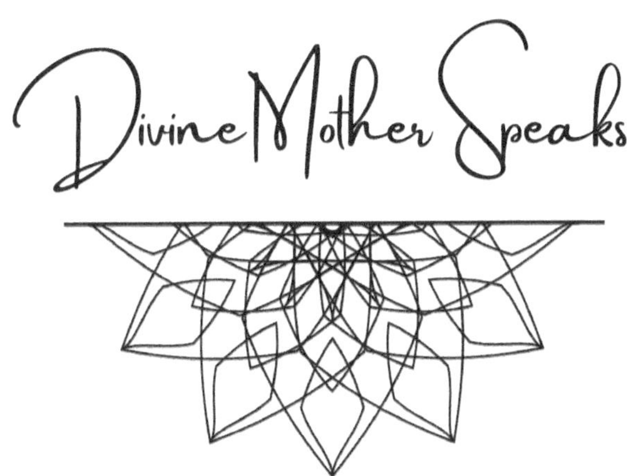

Divine Rebirth

Beloved Ones,

As an infinite Soul, you are in a constant state of rebirthing and bringing into being something new—forever creating and expanding your experience with Spirit. My message is that you are never ever alone in this process. However, it is clear that, at times, you feel as if you are.

Spirit loves to be a part of everything. However, the key is "be a part" of the equation. You are the other half. You are "One" with Spirit, not separate. Contributing does not always mean "doing" some sort of action. Co-creating through your inner Divine Wisdom also holds the space of love within your being to allow Spirit to do its part.

Divine Rebirth requires co-creation—we must work together. Birthing something new into existence—whether it be life or adventure—calls for a perfect balance of giving and receiving life-force energy. It must go both ways.

Rather than simply asking for what you desire, you must establish the ideal conditions for something to grow (Divine Manifestation). For example, you cannot expect a seed to flourish simply by putting it in a bowl and asking for a miracle. Co-create with the Universe by placing the seed into an environment where it will naturally thrive. Find some rich soil. Plant your seed of intention. Tend to it with love. Nurture it. Weed out all that is unnecessary so it has a clear path for growth. Then allow for the miracle of its life force to manifest into being.

Thought or prayer is your way of asking. Meditation, pausing, stillness, and silence allow you to see, hear, and know me, Divine Mother, and receive all necessary understandings to manifest your new beginning.

Where in your life are you floundering, desiring change but unsure or fearful about how to make it happen? Are you asking for Divine assistance and then allowing time and space for that assistance to come forward? Devoting time for silence and stillness is essential to see and find clarity in your request.

Love into your experience by embracing yourself and your adventures with your whole beautiful, sacred heart—leaving fear behind. Explore all things through the lens of pure, unconditional love. Your pure love and intention are the only way to manifest. The more you love into it, the deeper, more profound, and more expanded the vibration for change becomes.

Spirit is forever co-creating each and every experience. It is your choice to open yourself up to this ever-present Divine assistance.

With Loving Kindness,

Divine Mother

Chapter 3

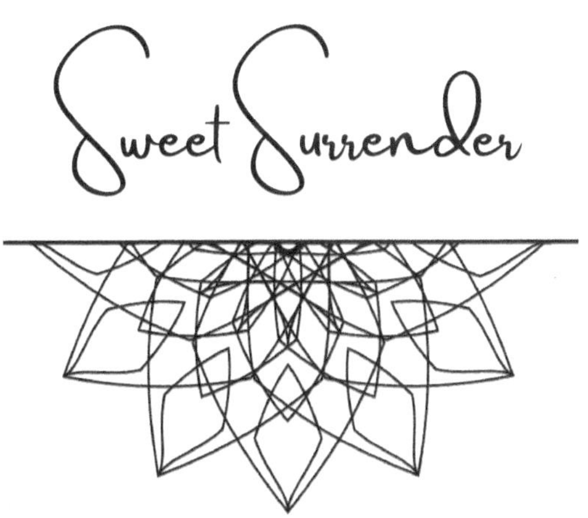

Third Sacred Truth
Divine Will

"Divine Will is to surrender ego into the Light of Divinity and the love of the Universe." –BT

To best understand the Third Sacred Truth, Divine Will, consider the phrase "Not my will, but Thine be done." Divine Will means emptying your mind of the lower ego and moving into Divine Knowingness. This beautiful Truth is about discerning when one's ego—specifically its fears, beliefs, and attachments—is superseding. When you are empowered by Divine Will, self-conflict transforms into purity and love for the world and yourself. And it is in such a transformation that we find freedom from myopic and egoic perspectives by scoping out to an expansive Spiritual path and surrendering all illusion of control.

Manipura (Muh-nee-poor-uh), located in the solar plexus, is the third chakra and Divine Will's energy center. This energy center's element is fire and is the home of "the self," or human identity, self-esteem, and self-worth. When living in alignment, this powerful energy center is also the seat of passion that propels us fearlessly forward. Working alongside the second chakra, Divine Will empowers us to take action on what we are most passionate about, powered with the wisdom and knowledge of our life's purpose. It inspires us to remember who we are and why we are here on this planet at this time in history. It also allows us to honor things as they are by recognizing the Divine Order in all things.

Sweet Surrender

"The only way to it is through it." You may be wondering where is "to it" and what do I mean by "getting through it"? "To it" is the other side of significant contrast or resistance in one's life. It's the place you could never imagine being—where things will never be the same. I do not suggest this is a bad thing because change profoundly expands one's experience and the lens through which we view our life. "Through it" is a place of momentous change and expanded self-awareness. Building on what we know about the Second Sacred Truth, Divine Rebirth, getting *through it* requires us to allow the flow of the experience rather than resisting the current. It has been my experience that the most peaceful way *through it* is by way of surrender.

Have you ever had an experience that has simply brought you to your knees? The pain of the event, at times, felt insurmountable. As human beings, everyone will be faced with a life-changing moment of contrast in which we are directly or indirectly impacted. It's part of living a full life. I have had a few times in my life in which my emotional pain was so devastating that I had no idea how to move forward. There was nothing anyone in my life could say or do to help me. It was just pure pain and suffering.

As the Dalai Lama puts it so beautifully, "Pain is inevitable. Suffering is optional." Over the past couple of years, this has been my biggest lesson and most difficult to interpret and integrate through my body's wisdom. Pain is a physical sensation, signaling something is off within the body. Suffering is our interpretation of that event which involves our thoughts, beliefs, or judgments as we reflect on our human experience of that pain. We can have both physical and emotional pain. On my journey, I have been stepping back and witnessing my pain as an observer to help distinguish when that pain crosses over into suffering. But how do I heal it once it has become suffering, based on my beliefs?

It became clear to me that I have an attachment to suffering, whether it be someone else's or my own. I desperately want to solve it and fix it. My higher wisdom knows that pain *is* inevitable; however, suffering doesn't have to be. Suffering is created by our desperate need and desire to *fight* the current and *fix* the situation that is causing the pain. By allowing suffering, we are subscribing to a myopic view of this life-changing and very human experience. In doing so, we so often miss the miracles that occur because we are desperately attached to fixing what *appears* to be broken. Our egos are constantly pinching off the flow of life by thinking rather than feeling our way through. Divine Mother teaches us to pause and observe an experience before making a judgment that anything needs to be "fixed." There is profound wisdom to be had when we observe through the lens of non-attachment and allow the heart to communicate truth while releasing fear-based comments from the ego.

We as humans have unlimited access to Divine Wisdom at all times. Our divinity has the ability to heal and move us through any and all things. What is required is recognizing the voice of the ego to "do something!" and instead to let go and let Spirit take over and light the path. This requires trust. Trust that if we release the stronghold we have around the situation and allow it to play out by using our Divine Guidance, we can love and ease ourselves through anything. We can then "*be* something" rather than "*do* something," permitting our higher self to guide us through the pain with compassion, patience, and kindness. There is truth in pain in that pain causes discomfort. It has been my experience that pain and discomfort are the biggest motivators for profound change.

The stories I am going to share with you continue to be an ongoing lesson for me as I navigate my strong desire to exert control. Control is simply our ego saying, "I am afraid." Looking at it this way makes it easy to find compassion for myself and my journey. When I am afraid, it's because I am not sure I will be able to handle the outcome, or I do not want to feel the worst-case scenario of this outcome. Being an empath, I cannot help but feel the pain and suffering of everyone around me, which drives me to find a solution to put an end to it.

When the "it" of getting *through it* is the loss of a loved one, it is difficult to imagine that this could be any sort of enlightened experience. When people are brought to their knees in grief, sadness, fear, and shame, getting *through it* means surrendering all control and folding into the core of our being to find ourselves again. A sense of humility goes along with true, authentic surrendering. That being said, some of the most significant acts have been accomplished, and some of the greatest potentials are realized when people are pushed so far into discomfort and the unknown. What we find is a strength we never knew we had. The ego has no place—in fact, the ego dies in the process.

Part I: Leo

My husband, two daughters, and I were returning from a week-long yoga retreat I had led in Costa Rica. Our flight landed late on the night of January 12th, 2020. We were tired but also rejuvenated from such a fun-filled time together. As we departed the plane, it was an abrupt shift from the tropical paradise we had just left to a good old Minnesota snowstorm. My sweet hubby went to go warm up the car as we awaited our luggage. After loading our bags into the car, we inched along the highway at about 25 mph—heading to drop my daughter, Lily, at her apartment. The snow was coming down hard, and the roads were icy. Lily asked if we all wanted to come in to say hello to her beloved pup, Dani. We chose to head back to our house because it was a minimum 45-minute drive, even in good driving conditions.

The entire way through the city, we followed a team of snowplows that led us safely but also delayed our return home even more. My daughter, Madeline, was at our house, awaiting our arrival. She wasn't able to go on the trip with us and was looking after our critters. My youngest daughter, Charlotte, was anxious to get home because her friend, Leo, was waiting at our house to say hello.

We live in a little river community on the outskirts of the Twin Cities. As we approached the final ten miles of winding road following the river, we found it had yet to be plowed. After 90 minutes of treacherous driving, we finally made it. Everyone jumped out of the car and ran inside to say hello. Madeline had fallen asleep in our bedroom, and she groggily came out. We shared all sorts of stories about our trip, and I unpacked the gifts we had gotten for her.

After several minutes of chatting, Charlotte suddenly remembered that Leo had come over and was waiting for her downstairs. We assumed he must have fallen asleep too. She ran down to say hello. (As I am preparing to write what comes next, my heart is racing, my hands are shaking, and tears are coming to my eyes. It's been over two years, and the experience is still so vivid and locked in my memory.)

From downstairs, I hear Charlotte scream, "Mom!!!" It was in a voice that I had never heard come out of her and also the kind of cry one never ever wants to hear. Everyone immediately knew that something was very wrong. I ran down as fast as I could. As I entered her room, I saw Leo slumped over on his side on Charlotte's bed. I quickly rolled him over and saw that his face and lips were blue. He was unresponsive and not breathing. It felt like time had stopped as I processed what I saw. My brain felt scrambled. I remember thinking, *No, this can't be what I am seeing.* I also remember thinking we need to call 911. My next very brief thought was second-guessing the severity of the scene.

Suddenly, my adrenaline kicked in and snapped me back into my body and into action. Everything went into auto-drive. I swiftly grabbed Leo by the shirt and hurled him to the ground. I told Charlotte to call 911 as I began administering CPR. I remember trying to match my compressions to the song "Stayin' Alive." While describing this experience, I am flashing back to a few years prior. I was sifting through my bedroom closet and came across an old at-home CPR instruction kit. My internal wisdom said, "Review this again, as you will be called to use it someday."

As I was administering mouth-to-mouth, there was a deep, guttural sound that came out of Leo after each breath. I tried to shift my focus and visualize that each breath I was giving was a breath of life, a breath of Spirit. But nothing I was doing was bringing him back to consciousness, and he still was not breathing. I felt almost certain that Leo began his journey through the tunnel of Light—he was on his journey home as his Spirit was leaving his body. We just needed to talk him back in. I continued to tell Leo, "Hang in there. There's so much to live for." I remember saying, "This will be a good story to tell tomorrow. I can't wait to hear where you went."

Charlotte kept coming in and out of the room. She was crying and also trying to stay calm. She amazed me with her strength that night. Madeline was standing outside, waiting to direct the EMTs when they arrived. Five minutes went by. Ten minutes. Twenty minutes. I kept yelling, "Where are they?" The 911 dispatcher said they were on the other side of Washington County and were navigating through the snowstorm. I thought, *Seriously? There's only one ambulance in this entire county that is available, and all the police just happen to be with it?*

I was beginning to fatigue. Joe asked if I needed him to step in, but I just couldn't stop my rhythm and let go. It was my only way to try to stay in control of what was happening. And I was desperately trying to stay in control. Strangely, I didn't feel panicked or anxious. I didn't pray, either. Instead, I had an intense determination to keep going and an underlying confidence that it would be okay.

Finally, at 29 minutes, the Sheriff and EMTs arrived. I know the exact time based on Madeline's call log. The EMTs ran downstairs and took over. They intubated him and kept saying his blood pressure was extremely low. The Sheriff came out to speak with each of us, asking if we had any idea if he had taken anything. I remembered Charlotte saying he had passed out on the hockey bus a couple of days prior. I wondered if he had a concussion. I also knew that he had a cashew allergy. Charlotte, being a vegan, had a lot of food in the house that was cashew based. The only thing I now find funny about that night was my obsession with his cashew allergy because I couldn't make sense of anything else.

As the event unfolded, we understood what the Sheriff wanted to know: if Leo was using drugs. Did we know anything about what he took? The Sheriff said the EMT administered two doses of Narcan, which revived Leo. Narcan is used to reverse the effects of an opioid overdose, namely slowed or stopped breathing. Leo had accidentally overdosed on an opioid laced with fentanyl. They found a portion of the pill in his wallet. He had only taken a sliver of the pill that night. Had he taken more, he would not have survived. After he was stable, Leo was transported to the hospital and released the next day.

None of us, including Charlotte, had any idea. Apparently, this drug of choice was an easy one to hide and is often called *the silent killer*. We later found out that this is why Leo passed out on the hockey bus as well. He had taken a sliver of this pill—not enough to stop his breathing. He regained consciousness on his own.

When I spoke with Leo after the event, I asked him what he needed. He wisely said, "Just time." Time does heal. It gives us space to allow emotions to surface and a moment to explore what we feel so we may gain perspective on the situation. It offers an insightful breath and the ability to see our way through.

After that night, I didn't feel all the grateful feelings one would think after such an event when the person actually survives. I didn't cry. I felt stuck in a loop of fear and anxiety, wondering if this would happen again. The words I used in my journal in the days following were, "I don't feel relief. I don't feel safe. I don't feel okay. It feels precarious, unsettled, and unfair. Unfair that we as humans have to navigate all of this shit and pain." What I didn't realize was that I was in shock and suppressing trauma.

In the following months, I found myself going about my day-to-day activities spiraling on the inside and acting as if nothing happened on the outside. The truth is there was rarely a moment that I didn't think about and relive that experience. Images of Leo continually flashed into my mind. I kept going over our steps prior to finding Leo unconscious, asking myself, *What if we stopped at Lily's to see her dog, Dani? What if Charlotte didn't go downstairs when she did? What if the snow slowed us down by just a few more minutes? What if I didn't remember how to administer CPR?* Every time I replay that night in my mind, my stress response is the same as if it were playing out in real-time. I kept telling myself, *But he's alive. This sweet kid is alive.*

At the time of the incident, I knew very little about opioids other than they were highly addictive. As I continued to process all that happened that night, I shared my experience in confidence with a friend who happened to be a cardiac nurse. She said Leo probably only had about 2–3 minutes before it was too late. She shared that opioids can interfere with receptors between the brain and heart, causing the heart rate to slow down and eventually stop. At some point, the brain is too starved of oxygen and will just quit communicating. I am so incredibly grateful I did not have this information while performing CPR. I cannot imagine the immense pressure that would have added to the situation. It was absolutely vital that I continued to have hope and not panic.

Part of understanding this story is knowing how much I care about that kid. Leo and Charlotte have been friends for years, and he feels like a part of the family. He practically lived at our house and continued to come over regularly. As the event in January became further and further away, Leo seemed to be doing pretty well. However, I was still hopeful he would go to treatment. My intuition knew this wasn't over.

As we approached March, spring break rolled around, and I went back to Costa Rica to look for more venues for a second yoga retreat. Leo, Charlotte, and a whole pile of their friends and chaperones went to Mexico. As I reflect on the situation, I realize that denial and wishful thinking became my way of coping. If you bury it deep enough, it isn't there, right? After all, Leo behaved just as he always had—as if all was well. He was functioning and going to school. He never looked under the influence. He was his happy, joyful, engaging self every time I saw him. We had a very long conversation about the incident, and he promised me that if he felt like he wanted to use again, he *for sure* would get help.

Part II: Tyler

Meet Tyler. My daughter, Lily, would describe him as *bigger* than life! He was her best friend. All of my girls loved him dearly. His laugh was this funny kind of infectious giggle. He had an unbelievable smile that made everyone feel like life was pretty good. Lily said that whenever she and Tyler would arrive at a party together, it felt like she was accompanied by a celebrity. As they walked through the crowd, she thought to herself, *That's right, I'm here with Tyler.* When in need, Tyler and Lily showed up for each other no matter the time, place, or circumstance. She could share anything and everything with him. He wasn't full of advice, just an open mind and expansive heart. He was her person, and she was that for him as well. She told me once that she felt like he looked at her as if she was perfect, and he unconditionally accepted every part of who she was—no matter what. They never dated, which made their relationship easy and uncomplicated.

So I will pick up my story where I left off with Leo, as these two experiences intertwine. It is worth saying that the two of them knew of each other but had not spent time together. My hope, as you read on, is that you will find compassion over judgment. I chose to write this book to show that everyone has their own struggles and also, maybe, more importantly, this section reveals how prevalent the opioid and fentanyl crisis is in this country––most especially among our youth and young adults.

It was March 2020, and the world was going into lockdown due to Covid. Tyler had just survived his second overdose of that year, and Lily had asked if I would meet with him. After reaching out to Tyler, we decided to take a walk together. We met at my house after work and headed down towards the river. It was a warm March evening as the sun was beginning to set. We sat down at the marina, our feet dangling just above the water. We talked about anything and everything. For some reason, it didn't feel like a heavy conversation, given the circumstances. It was just an honest exchange about where he was in his life and how his actions had impacted his family, friends, and himself. He shared what had happened with the overdose and the guilt he felt for putting all of his loved ones through it. I could feel he was just tired of living with the burden of substance use disorder and was ready to surrender. We discussed going to inpatient treatment as an option, and he was open to exploring it. As the sun had almost set and the wind picked up, we decided to make our way back to the house.

When we got back, Tyler hugged me and headed home to discuss his next steps with his family. One thing about

Tyler and Leo is that they both give the most amazing hugs. I can always tell how open someone's heart is by the intensity of their hug—with outstretched arms and a big squeeze that lasts until you can feel hearts exchanging love. I can't tell you how much these two kids mean to me.

About a week after our talk, Tyler was making plans to check into Hazelden Treatment Center. Coincidentally, Leo also chose to enter a program with Hazelden. Since Leo was still a minor, he was at a different facility. I was relieved that both of them were getting the care they needed. I was unaware until months later that Leo had also accidentally overdosed a second time in March.

Because we were in unprecedented times due to the Covid epidemic, in-person treatment was mostly virtual. All therapy sessions were done via Zoom. The group sessions were on pause. Understandably, it was difficult for both Leo and Tyler to feel very engaged with their programs. Tyler remained in the program for about three weeks, and Leo for a little over a month.

After Tyler left treatment, we continued to do our "walk and talks." On one of our walks, I came up with a proposition for him. I had just begun a 200-hour yoga teacher training program that had been interrupted by the lockdown. We were going to begin to meet again in person, and I asked Tyler if he would like to join the group. He could take the course for free in exchange for help with our house remodel. I thought this might be a wonderful fit because the foundation of my yoga teacher training is about finding and living joyfully in one's purpose through the healing aspects of yoga. The bonus is that you also graduate with the skills to be an awesome yoga instructor. Tyler took me up on my proposal, and I introduced him to my class the following weekend.

Because of this new setup, I had the privilege of seeing Tyler a couple of evenings a week and most weekends, either at my house or at class. Throughout the spring and summer, he seemed to be thriving. He showed up on time and prepared for every class. At the end of each class, he stayed behind to help me clean up and walk me to my car. He'd hug me with that big bear hug and say, "I love you, Suzy." Then off he'd go on his excruciatingly loud Harley motorcycle.

When July rolled around, we were three-quarters of the way through the program. We met on Friday night to begin our weekend intensive. Tyler was super engaged. He shared with the class his experience teaching a full yoga class to his mom and girlfriend earlier in the week. He expressed how much fun they had together. He also shared that teaching yoga was what he wanted to do with his life. He expanded on that by sharing his dream to open a yoga retreat center on the family land up north. On our break, he told me about an amazing day with Lily. They spent the entire day lying out in the grass at his parent's lake home, talking about nothing and everything. It sounded just perfect. I thought how lucky the two of them were to have such an extraordinary friendship. All of his relationships seemed to be in a perfect place.

As our Friday night was coming to a close, I said goodbye to the class. Tyler helped me clean up and walked me to my car. For the first time, he didn't hug me goodbye. I was feeling a bit cautious about Covid that night and thought maybe it was better that way. But he also didn't say I love you either. At the time, I didn't make much of it other than thinking he must be preoccupied. My biggest regret is that I didn't say it either. I was also in a distracted mood. It was late, and I was tired and just wanted to get home.

I got into my car, facing Tyler and his motorcycle on the opposite side of the street. I watched him get on his bike and look at his phone for a while. My first thought was that I should wait and make sure he gets off okay. I was famished after teaching all night and decided to head out. I drove past him and waved goodbye.

The following day I received a call from Tyler's girlfriend. Her voice was trembling, and I knew in that moment that this was the call I prayed I would never receive. I so badly wanted to stop her from continuing. She said Tyler was found dead in his parent's home due to an accidental drug overdose. I just stood there in utter disbelief. Not even 24 hours prior, he was so joyful and enthusiastic, planning out his future. He had come so far.

As I hung up the phone, this horrible feeling came over me. I was the last person to see him, or so I thought. I didn't hug him, and I didn't say, "I love you." I broke the one rule I preached to my girls throughout their lives. "Whenever you leave each other, be sure to say, 'I love you,' as you never know when you will see them again." Ughhh. I don't know how to describe how this felt other than I failed him. I felt like I should have seen this coming. I should have noticed the cues. How in the world did I not intuit this situation? And now I had to tell my daughter, Lily, that her very best friend in the whole world had died.

That Saturday, Lily was at a friend's cabin. I was just praying she didn't receive the news via social media or some random phone call or text. We were watching her dog, Dani, so I sent her a message asking if she could come home early. I told her Dani seemed out of sorts and missed her. She responded and said she'd head home and be back by early evening.

My heart. Oh, my heart. I just couldn't even think about how I was going to tell her this news. I spent the day nervously pacing about and crying. Hours went by when I heard her car pull up. I let Dani go out to greet her. She came inside, and I thought I was going to throw up. She was standing by the fridge and asked what was wrong. I told her, "Honey, I'm so sorry. Tyler died today from an accidental overdose." She screamed and dropped to the floor. She just kept saying, "No, no, no, no, no!" It was all just so awful and the most difficult thing I have ever had to say. It was another punch in the gut. I knew there was nothing I could do to take this pain away.

The words "What if?" continually replay in my mind. What if I had looked him in the eyes before we parted ways? What if I had hugged him? I am an intuitive healer! How did I miss the signs? Was he planning on doing this before he got on his bike that Friday night? It turns out that his dealer and childhood friend had been reaching out for months, trying to get him to use with him again. Prior to this day, Tyler had responded each time by saying, "Nope, I'm sober now, and I'm living a clean life." We'll never know why he chose this time to accept—the answers to all these questions left with Tyler.

Because I spent so much time with Tyler in the final months of his life, I felt incredibly responsible for him. And because these two kids, Leo and Tyler, were living seemingly parallel lives until that awful day in July, I felt even more manic about making sure Leo stayed sober and, more importantly, alive.

Thus began a deep internal spiraling. My whole foundation got knocked off its footing. I had deep, deep grief and trauma all twisted up in my gut from these experiences. Everything in me recognized how unhealthy this was, but I just could not step around my ego as it was screaming, "You CANNOT allow this to happen again!" A switch flipped on inside of me that I didn't know how to turn off. From that day forward, I made it my mission that Leo would not see the same fate as Tyler. The word *CONTROL* was my battle cry. I absolutely could not and would not go through this pain again!

Shortly after Tyler died, Charlotte and Leo chose to go their separate ways. Not being able to see Leo regularly just triggered my fears even more. In the fall of 2020, Leo accidentally overdosed a third time. His Mom called me to share the news. I met with him, and we went for a walk in the woods, then sat by the river. He burrowed his head in his hands and cried. He looked so broken and discouraged. All I wanted was to take the pain and opioid addiction away. I could do neither of those things. We sat in silence for quite a while. I was trying to hold the space for him to be whatever he needed to be at that moment.

We talked about treatment. He was not interested in going back. We talked about getting a sponsor and finding group meetings. Everything was still virtual. None of the steps to help him to get healthy seemed to inspire him. I asked him what he needed. His response was again, "Just time." We agreed to meet regularly and just go for walks and talk.

On one of our walks, I asked if he would get a shot that specifically helps people with opioid use disorder (OUD) not feel the high should they decide to use again. Some experts say it is one of the best ways to deter persons with OUD from using and keeps them alive. We went around and around about this because he didn't see the value. I stopped on the path and began to sob, slowly becoming unglued. He hugged me. I told him I just could not continue to support him if he wasn't going to use this tool. It was breaking me. I begged him to do this for me. And by the end of the walk, he agreed.

After I got home, I knew this wasn't how it worked. He cannot do this for me. Whatever he does has to be for himself. I began to recognize that I was losing a part of myself. I also noticed a pattern when I inserted the word "I" into his recovery. "I" could not go through this again. "I" could not tolerate the pain and suffering. The bottom line is that his recovery *had* to be about him. I also recognized that I have a pretty serious issue with suffering. More specifically, watching people suffer. I want to fix it because, being an empath, *I* am suffering right along with them. Fixing someone else's problem may feel better to me in the short term. Still, I realized by stepping in, I am robbing that person, specifically Leo, of a life-changing, empowering experience to do it himself. In other words, I am saying, "Because of my overwhelming fear, I don't trust you to do this yourself, so I will take over." All parents out there, if you are inserting yourself into your child's or anyone's decision-making, re-read that last statement. Taking control away disempowers the other person. By saying, "I think you should..." is saying, "I know better." It takes away their ability and opportunity to navigate according to their own inner wisdom. Spirit gives us the freedom of choice and will never step in and take that away. Spirit may show us signs to help guide our decisions, but will never, ever intercede and make them for us. Both Leo and Tyler are very wise individuals, and only their souls know the wisdom of their paths.

Knowing that my fear was steering the ship was one thing. Now it was time to integrate this understanding, step back, and trust Leo. My heart and my truth understood it was not my fault Tyler died, and that I had any power to keep Leo alive. But my ego had been ruthlessly attached to a place of survival for myself and them. As I reflect on my feelings and actions, I am finding compassion for myself. I was so profoundly sad, angry, and heartbroken. There were just so many maternal emotions that I had for these two. I simply didn't know how to reconcile any of it.

The Gift In Surrender

As I observed my mental and emotional state, it was obvious that I had been battling depression since the summer of 2020. I no longer had the capacity to hold everything together. The imagery I received was of me juggling balls. I can manage it at first, but then someone keeps throwing more balls into my act. I begin to lose one and quickly pick up another. I lose a few more and desperately try to maintain the ones I still have going. It's a very manic feeling between being in perfect control and then hopelessly losing everything. When I get to the point of total exhaustion and finally let all the balls drop, that is the moment of surrender. I finally get to a place where I don't have any more reserve to be able to attach to an outcome. When I allow myself to drop all the balls, my arms are free to open up, and I begin to expand my outlook and recognize that I never truly had control in the first place.

It was at this point that I sat down and prayed—and prayed and prayed and prayed and prayed. I prayed for help in surrendering this burden. I had to face the pain and trauma I experienced with Leo and Tyler and own it. Leo had to face his opioid use disorder and own it according to his inner guidance.

My decision to finally surrender broke the spell. It unlocked something in me that allowed for healing to begin. It allowed my ego to let go of the situation that was not mine to fix in the first place. I opened my hands and let Leo and Tyler go. I opened my heart and allowed Spirit to come in and heal.

Throughout the past three years, I continually go into meditation and ask for help and guidance with my grieving and trauma. What I know is that Leo and Tyler are two amazing teachers in my life. They each gave me the gift of a deeper understanding about pain vs. suffering, control vs. surrendering, and ego vs. Divine Will. I am grateful and am humbly doing my work to *Stand in My Truth* and find peace.

– Oh, and Leo has been opioid-free for almost three years now. His internal wisdom and choice not to take that monthly shot empowered him to realize he has the resources to manage his OUD without the need for another drug. Now, as a twenty-year-old, he got his real estate license and just purchased a beautiful farmhouse overlooking the St. Croix River Valley, which he is personally renovating. We still meet for walks, and I am greeted each time with his amazing hug.

– And Tyler...I still feel his presence often. His magnificent Spirit shows up in nature. His mom says that when she is thinking of him, she often sees an eagle flying overhead. On the day of his celebration of life, there was an eagle that kept watch over all of us while we honored his sweet soul. There's a peacefulness knowing that Tyler made his way home.

Help In Healing Through Divine Will

Sometimes it seems nearly impossible to release the outcome of a situation—especially if it is a life-or-death scenario. It feels unimaginable to surrender rather than fight. I would love for you to take a moment and consider the vibration of fighting, controlling, and attaching to certain outcomes. It feels like grasping a bar of wet soap. There's so much effort to control it from slipping out of your hand rather than gently allowing it to sit in your palm. Inevitably, the harder you squeeze, the more likely you are to lose it.

I find it interesting how we speak about illness, for example, *fighting* cancer or any sort of substance use disorder. I'm not suggesting just sitting back and doing nothing about it. I am suggesting to consider how we frame it in our minds and hearts. What if we *loved* into our situation and *loved* into our body rather than fought against it? After all, cancer is something our body creates. What if we spoke gently and lovingly to ourselves? The vibration is entirely different. When we allow rather than fight, we are in a flow, and the resistance fades away. We can still take all of the steps we feel necessary to heal the issue, but it is done in a loving way. The body will accept that love, find more ease, and assist in its own healing.

As you have heard from my example, it took me over a year to finally surrender. Mostly because I didn't know how to let go. I felt like I would be abandoning Leo. At one point, I even considered stepping back for my own mental health. Divine Mother came to me during meditation and said,

"You do not need to walk away from Leo; you simply need to walk away from your fear. I am not asking you to give up hope. I am asking you to give up control."

This required trust—trust that the situation is under the perfect Divine Guidance. That's when I literally got down on my knees, placed my forehead on the floor, and opened up my hands. My prayer went something like this:

I am in so much pain. I have no idea how to make this situation better. I feel desperate. I feel lost. I feel abandoned. I feel angry. I have nowhere to turn. In this desperate moment, I surrender all of these emotions. I lay my burdens down and ask for peace in my heart and for guidance to see this situation through. Help me to love into this and know that I am not alone. Great Spirit, grant me the serenity to accept the things I cannot change, courage to change the things I can, and the wisdom to know the difference.

And then I just lay there and cried like a baby. Everything spilled out of me until there was nothing left but remarkable stillness. I felt cradled in an indescribable light.

What burdens are you carrying around? Visualize that bar of soap or, better yet, carrying a backpack full of large rocks. Each rock represents an attachment or burden you have been carrying around and trying to control. That backpack gets heavy and exhausting to drag around. At some point, the weight of the backpack and your burdens will become unmanageable, putting your joy and health at risk.

- I invite you to take inventory of your life and recognize how full your backpack is or how many *bars of soap* you are clenching in your fist.
- Validate your feelings and struggles by giving each burden a name.
- Recognize what is your responsibility and what requires your attention.
- Then send up a prayer asking for help in releasing your egoic attachments.
- Surrender, surrender, surrender.
- Pause and be still.

- Allow and love into it rather than fight.
- Finally, awaken to your beautiful Divine Will (*Not my will, but Thine be done*) as your personal guide through it.

Divine Will Affirmation

"I am the Light of Divine Will. Through this Sacred Truth, I am able to supersede my ego and surrender to the wisdom of my Divinity, allowing me to feel the beauty, bliss, and perfection in all things."

Journaling Questions

- Are you feeling pain, or is it suffering?
- What are you attached to that is causing this suffering? An attachment isn't a fact or truth; it is a belief system that can create a false and weakened sense of Self.
- What is going on in your life that you feel you need to control?
- How can you scope out or step back from the situation and view the bigger picture as an observer rather than a participant?
- How can you see beauty through the pain?
- What changes are going on in your life that you may be resisting?

- How do you feel about surrendering what you cannot change?
- What are you trying to fix?
- How does it feel to allow the situation to be just as it is?
- Even better, can you look at the situation, whether it be a person or circumstance, as having its own Divine Plan/Wisdom?

Yoga & Meditation

Our yoga practice will be a bit fiery, with intense breathwork and many twists and compressions to rinse and release unnecessary emotions. It will end with a blissful series of surrendering postures leading to a restorative meditation in which I will prompt you to name, validate, and relinquish your burdens. To access your classes, scan the QR code or visit the link.

https://bit.ly/3W3sueX

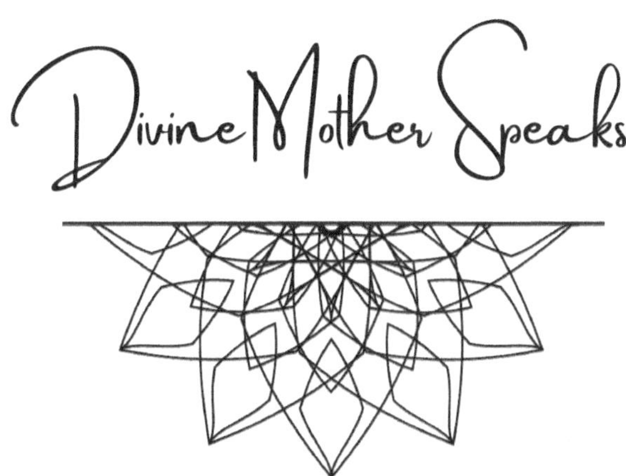

Divine Will

Beloved Ones,

When you are speaking to me, please know that I am everywhere at all times. You can access me in the forest, your dreams, and even the grocery store. I am everywhere, and I am all things.

When you consider Divine Will, I ask that you pause when your vibration is lower and take the time to release that which is negative because I cannot come down to that vibration. You must surrender what you are holding on to and allow your vibration to neutralize from frustrations, grief, or whatever is negatively impacting your life.

I often witness human experiences in which one spirals over and over with the same issues. There are thoughts or prayers sent, but no change occurs. The reason is that fear creates control. And control pinches off the flow of life. Thus, the pattern repeats itself.

Fear is a natural part of being human. Surrendering the fear into Divine Will expands the view, and you recognize that you do not need to walk the journey alone.

Fear shadows the truth and your ability to see the situation clearly. Surrendering into Divine Will allows the Light to shine on the situation and cracks the door for change to come in.

I am requesting that you trust the journey. I honor all of your emotions and am holding the space for you to offer them up. Walking through the fear is a process not to be judged by how long it takes or how it takes place.

Once you relinquish these burdens from your purest heart, it is then that I can come in to assist you with whatever you desire. Surrendering is as simple as sending a heartfelt thought or a prayer. It could be something like this.

"I am ready to surrender these feelings and experiences that keep me from

knowing joy, peace, and abundance. I request your help."

That is all it takes.

You will find serenity when you open your hands to receive and allow the Light to come in. And with serenity comes clarity. And with clarity comes the beginning of the resolution you are looking for. Please understand you are never alone—ever. I observe your struggles and always send support and love. Always.

With Loving Kindness,

Divine Mother

PART II

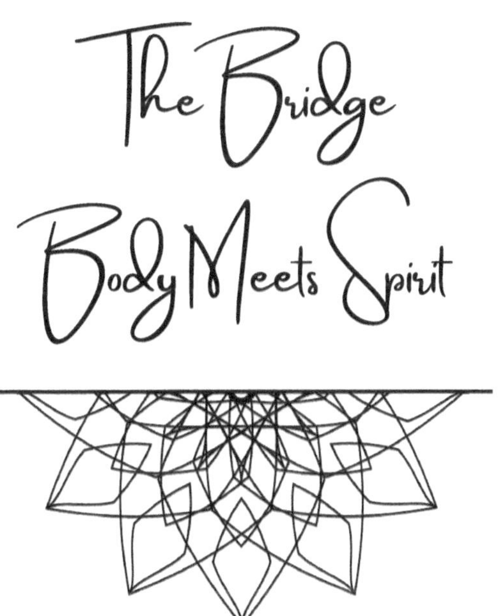

As we move into chapter four and explore the Heart Center, I'll describe how this energy center bridges our human experiences with our Spiritual experiences. My goal in this chapter is to help you understand how to communicate through the unconditional love of the heart.

Chapter 4

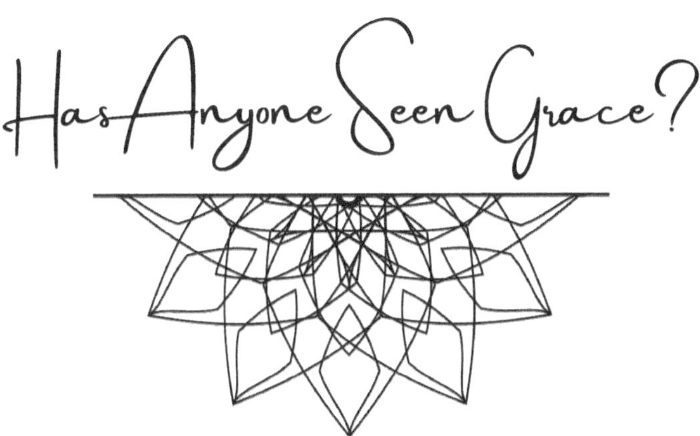

Fourth Sacred Truth
Divine Love

The Fourth Sacred Truth, Divine Love, is our moral and Spiritual compass. Therefore, we must be sure that all of our intentions are firmly rooted and aligned with this Sacred Truth. Holding this intention moves us beyond egoic will and into a place of humble and blessed devotion to our sacred divinity. Our Spiritual lesson from The Fourth Sacred Truth teaches us how to act from a place of pure compassion and love. Divine Love is the source of a deep and profound inner knowingness that is not expressed through words. It allows us to experience unconditional love and feel our connection to all things. Once we are familiar with the vibration of love, we can immediately feel when our thoughts, actions, and deeds are out of attunement and are able to adjust our course.

Divine Love coincides with the fourth chakra called the Anahata (Unn-ah-huh-tah) or heart chakra and is located behind and just to the right of our physical heart. The element associated with the heart chakra is air. The heart center mediates or bridges our body and Spirit. The divinity within our heart center does not see the body and the Spirit as separate. Instead, it integrates them into one harmonious vibration of giving and receiving. Divine Loving Wisdom lives deep within your beautiful heart and is the home of Spirit. You are able to find the answers and, more importantly, the truth to absolutely everything if you allow your heart to speak. The love language of your heart knows no fear. It knows no shame. It knows no pity or guilt. The language of your heart speaks only through compassion, peace, bliss, harmony, understanding, empathy, clarity, purity, unity, kindness, forgiveness, and of course, love. I encourage you to step around the ego and the intellectual mind and listen. Just listen to the wisdom of your heart.

My Story of Love

The story I am about to share stretched my heart to its emotional limits until it finally broke apart. Only then did I find grace and remember that I *am* love. Here is my story.

My dad opened my eyes daily to the miracles that are all around us. As a kid, I remember looking out the kitchen window with him on a terribly cold January day. We noticed the chickadees out in a tree. I felt sorry for the birds, but he was in awe about how they were perfectly equipped to survive even the harshest winters. He said, "This was just another miracle in this beautiful Divine plan."

As a self-taught pianist, my dad could play by ear. To unwind after work, he would sit down and play the piano while my mom made dinner. My favorite memories from childhood are the times I spent dancing in the living room to his music. As soon as his car drove up, I would run up and get my dance partner, Henry, a beloved stuffed dog. I'd also throw on one of my mom's flowy flowered nightgowns, which would poof out as I spun around. My dad was born in 1928 and loved to unleash a little boogie-woogie music of the 1930s and '40s. We had a bay window in our living room, so at night, I could see my reflection in all of the windows. It looked like there was a party of about 20 people, all dancing in synchronicity. Henry and all of our other dance partners would jump around that living room as long as he kept playing. When it was time for dinner, my dad would end our dance party with my favorite song, "Somewhere Over The Rainbow," from *The Wizard of Oz*. The movie scared the bejeebers out of me, but that song will always remind me of him and our special time together.

On hot summer nights, while my brother and I were taking a bath and getting ready for bed, my dad often drove to our local Bridgeman's ice cream and got four butter brickle ice cream cones. They'd put them in some sort of carrier, and he'd drive all the way home holding the cones out the window with ice cream running down his arm. This was a messy but wonderful memory.

I had so much in common with my dad, and we shared similar hobbies. My dad and I both loved to swim, and we also loved to paint and draw. When it came to my art, he was my biggest fan. As I got into high school and college, that is where I directed my studies. He once told me, "Never give up your art, Honey. That will be something you will enjoy for your entire life." He was right. Drawing and painting have continued to be a source of joy and a meditative escape for me.

I often think about my wedding day and holding my dad's hand while he walked me down the aisle. Holding his sweet soft hand calmed my nerves, and his gentle voice reassured me. When we got to the altar, there were tears in his eyes. As he handed me off to my soon-to-be husband, Joe, he said in a shaky voice, "Take care of her."

While I was in labor with my first daughter, Madeline, my mom and dad came to the hospital to see how I was doing. I remember hearing the sound of my mom's voice down the hall. It made me cry with relief as my labor was intensifying. They had only meant to stop in briefly, but ten hours later, my dad captured a phenomenal photo of Madeline's very first breath. People often ask if having my dad in the delivery room felt weird. My modest Catholic dad sat by my head at the top of the bed and was in awe of the entire experience. Having adopted his children, he had never witnessed a birth before. So having him there felt like the most natural thing in the world.

When I was in my 30s, my dad began to stumble frequently, having trouble picking up his foot. Soon after, he started to lose feeling in his feet. His speech became slurred until it became difficult to understand his words.

After many doctor visits, we found ourselves physically exhausted, emotionally depleted, and waiting in a small neurologist's office at The Mayo Clinic in Rochester, Minnesota. My dad had been through three full days of testing. Throughout the testing—both cognitive and physical—my dad looked at me with his sweet, sweet expression. "Did I pass?" he would ask. "Did I do okay?" It broke my heart because I knew this was not a situation in which passing or doing well would matter.

The doctor came in. For the life of me, I can't remember anything about him. I only recall him saying, "Although there are no definitive tests, we feel certain that John has ALS (Lou Gehrig's Disease)." The rest is a blur. I took in a deep breath and looked at my mom and then my dad. He didn't understand the diagnosis. He thought if he worked hard enough that he would get better. I felt the tears welling up in my eyes. I knew if I exhaled, it would be with loud sobs.

I stepped out of the doctor's office so I wouldn't upset my dad. My world was imploding as I walked with no direction. I found myself in the large atrium of one of the main buildings. There were people from across the world having all sorts of experiences—doctors, nurses, patients, families, children. There was a piano player. Kids were dancing. Some were singing. It was a surreal taste of Disneyland in the middle of a hospital. I sat by an atrium window and watched the strange scene unfold in front of me. I couldn't move or breathe. I wasn't sure how to process my dad's diagnosis. I didn't feel connected to my body. I felt like I was placed in the middle of a tornado as I watched everything swirl around me. I came back to earth while calling my husband, telling him the news. The experience became real as the words left my mouth, "My dad is dying—he has ALS."

At that moment, I realized there is no such thing as *doing well in life.* We are here to experience each moment for what it brings—whether it be love, joy, distress, pain, support, or all the above. We are here to richly experience and share in each moment, no matter the circumstance or the outcome.

During this journey, I had two pivotal experiences with my dad. The first occurred while taking my dad out for a walk around the neighborhood in his wheelchair. My dad had such a peaceful and joyful disposition. Whenever I entered the door at his care facility for a visit, he would clap his hands, and his eyes and mouth would open in a joyful expression. Smiling, he'd mouth the words, "Oh my!" He'd do the same when they offered him ice cream. When asked how he was doing, he'd give the thumbs-up sign, followed by a "Pretty good."

However, on this particular day, he was aggressive and frustrated. Halfway around the block, he began to direct angry noises at me because he had lost his ability to speak coherently. He was motioning that he wanted to turn around and go back.

I eased his wheelchair around to face me. We were in the middle of the street. I asked him, "Dad, are you afraid?" I got a nod. I then asked, "Are you afraid to die?" Tears flowed down his face, and he mouthed the word, "Yes." He began to sob. I placed one hand on his heart and held his hand with the other. I told him, "I am going to walk through this with you. You are not on this journey alone. I will be with you on this side, holding your hand until you are ready to cross over and take the hand of the Creator." Did those words come from me, or were those the words of Divine Inspiration? Yes. Yes, to both.

As I write these words, my dog, Penny, pulls on my shirt. Seeing that I am sad, she's looking at me as if to say, "I am here. See me. See my support and unconditional love." My other dog, Winnie, walked over to offer her stuffed animal, Bob, with the same expression. Support shows up in many different forms—One *being*, whether human or animal, feeling and responding to the vibration of another. This is one of those miracles my dad told me to watch for.

The second pivotal moment occurred when I was lying with my dad in his bed at the hospice home. His ability to speak had long since left him. However, that didn't stop him from chattering all day and especially all night. He'd go on and on about something and then turn to me, "Hmm?" as if to ask what I thought. I had no answer because I hadn't the faintest idea of what he said. I'd do my best to respond, and he'd shrug his shoulders, satisfied with my answer, and continue the conversation.

The process of getting him to sleep was similar to a young child who wanted to stay up as late as possible. One night, I placed my hand on his heart to settle him. With my hand upon his heart, I began to understand what he was trying to say. Eventually, I knew exactly what he was communicating. We began to speak to each other through our hearts and discovered a new language between us. I'd feel his emotions and would send back a response. No words were uttered or necessary. Eventually, he would settle and drift off to sleep, content with our communication. Our souls learned the process of enlightened communication—a soul conversation. It was beautiful.

As my dad was going through the final stages of ALS, I remember driving around feeling like I just needed to exhale. I felt like there was a belt around my chest that just kept squeezing me tighter and tighter the longer he suffered and remained in his body. I remember driving home from our visits and visualizing his transition. I would get this feeling in the pit of my stomach and a tightening in my throat. It was absolute resistance to facing my dad's inevitable journey.

On the evening of April 30th, I was in my dad's hospice room with his nurse, Deb. She and her husband, Dan, had been our saving grace throughout my dad's stay in hospice. She lovingly nicknamed my dad Johnny. As we were getting Johnny ready for bed, he suddenly got violently ill all over the three of us. Our strange reaction was laughter. We looked at each other with an expression of, "I have no idea what to do right now." After five years of this, the idea of anything being gross at this point didn't even register.

What I knew in my heart was this evening was the beginning of his transition. He never ate or drank after that day. I remember feeling relief, among all other emotions, that this five-year journey was coming to an end. Strangely, one thing I didn't feel that night was self-judgment about my emotions. I was simply too exhausted and was able to let it go.

As the days went by, my dad got weaker and weaker. We brought the priest in for my dad's last rites. On that day, it's like he had a second wind. He was alert and participated in the prayers. He even pretended to do pull-ups on the hospital bar he once used to assist himself out of bed. I was mentally and emotionally preparing for his transition, and on this day, he looked as if he was going to get back out of bed and play the piano. I realized this instigated a false sense of hope—one I had felt many times throughout this experience. It also triggered some anger. I absolutely couldn't see myself going back and tightening that belt around my chest another notch. Not another inhale. I remember speaking very angrily to Spirit, asking why this experience felt so cruel.

My dad's second wind only lasted a few hours. The gift in these few hours is that he was aware enough to receive and respond through the expression on his face to any final words we needed to say. As he began to fade back out, the angels came in. He was no longer present to me but was reaching and holding his hands out with a look of pure innocence and curiosity, just like a child. The veil was being lifted. He began his communication and rebirth with the other side. He began his journey home.

In the final couple of days, he spiked a high temperature. No longer conscious, he was lying with only a sheet draped over his lower body and his legs hanging out. He was so, so thin. It was day eleven without food or water. We all knew that it would be soon. My mom, brother, hubby Joe and my girls were all there. Joe and the girls wanted to give us some privacy and said their goodbyes. I'll never forget Joe's last words to my dad. He leaned in, gave him a kiss on the head, and whispered, "Don't worry, John, I'll take care of her."

Oh! My heart! I cannot tell you how much that meant to me that my husband remembered what my dad had asked of him when he handed me over to Joe on our wedding day. I'm certain those words brought considerable comfort to my dad, allowing him to transition more peacefully.

After they left, I created a bed on the floor and got comfortable for a long night ahead. My brother stood up and said, "Well, I think I am going to go." Shortly after that, my mom said she thought she would also head home.

I stood up in absolute disbelief. We had come this far; everyone knew we were down to the final hours. We were all incredibly exhausted, but I felt I *should* stay. I fought with myself because I promised to walk him through his transition. In hindsight, my mom and brother clearly understood something I did not.

As I sat there, the wisdom of my heart spoke. I knew I needed to let him go, or he would continue to hold on and suffer. It was my time to find grace for myself, surrender what I thought I *should* do, and listen to my dad's heart— what I knew he truly desired. He needed me to say goodbye and go.

My mom and brother said their heartfelt goodbyes and stepped out of the room. I was all alone with him. Through lots of tears, I held his face in my hands, kissed him on his sweet bald head, and said, "I love you, I love you, I love you, I love you." Then I walked out the door.

This was the hardest thing I have ever had to do. It triggered every emotion in me. My ego kept shouting, "You are abandoning him when he needs you the most! You are abandoning him! You promised him you would be there. What are you doing????" Regardless of what my ego was expressing, I summoned up the courage, got in my car, and drove away.

It was late when I arrived home, and I quietly crawled into bed. I was in a strange wake/sleep state all night. I had the phone beside me. The nurse promised someone would call if anything happened. At about 4 a.m., something nudged me fully awake. I immediately called hospice. The young aide, who couldn't have been more than twenty years old, anxiously answered the phone. She told me he had just passed. She slipped out for two minutes to go to the bathroom, and he chose that moment of silence to leave.

Strangely, I didn't cry when I heard the news. I just got up and began doing laundry. I didn't call my brother or mom because, for some reason, I didn't want to wake them up. I sat in the stillness of dawn and felt this weird sense of calm. It was over. What I had feared the most had happened. I was through it. I surrendered and let him go. The tight belt around my chest released, and I could breathe again. For a few short moments, I felt peace.

While sitting here, reflecting on that time, I can faintly hear "Somewhere Over The Rainbow" playing in my husband's office downstairs. This brings me right back into my dad's hospice room as if no time had passed. Tears flow down my cheeks. It's not because I wish he were back again. It's because I am looking at myself, my dad, and my experience during that time with such compassion. I was a 43-year-old woman with three kids of my own. I guess it doesn't matter how old you are when a parent dies. For me, there was still a little girl saying goodbye to her dad.

The Gift

On the first Christmas after my dad transitioned, I had an experience that allowed me to see how my body was holding on to the grief. It was a beautiful day. The sun was shining, and we had just gotten a fresh snowfall. So my family decided to go sledding. The five of us, plus our dog, Winnie, got all bundled up and trudged our way over to the sledding hill. After a few runs, my girls wanted to do the family sled. So three of us piled on, with me in the middle, and down we went. We picked up quite a bit of speed with my dog Winnie racing beside us.

As we neared the bottom of the hill, we went over a very small jump. It was just enough to lift me off the sled and slam me back down. Having broken my tailbone as a child, I immediately knew something wasn't right. When we got down to the bottom, everyone could tell I had gotten hurt. As they came over to help me, I yelled, "Nobody touch me! I think I broke something." I lay in the snow for a while until the intensity lessened. I rolled onto my side and wiggled my way back up to standing. I looked up the steep hill, knowing I had to waddle myself to the top somehow. It took a while, but I made it up the hill and back home. I iced my bum and went on to Christmas dinner at my in-laws' house. When I couldn't sit down without excruciating pain, I knew I had to get it checked out. It turned out I broke my sacrum in three places.

After a few months of discomfort, the break repaired itself, but the pain was still pretty significant. I decided to do some yoga therapy to loosen up the muscles supporting my sacrum. The instructor guided me through some gentle movements. She put me into a restorative pose and left the room for me to relax. As I was lying there, I found myself slipping into an altered state. It was like I had entered a time warp. I was back at the sledding hill where the incident occurred. Only this time, everything showed up in hyper colors and a sort of magnified awareness. The entire experience occurred in slow motion. As we began our descent down the hill, I could see clear details of Winnie's face as she was running beside me. I saw each individual snowflake floating in the air as they caught the sunlight and radiated a diamond-like rainbow ray of light. As I passed by my daughter, Lily, I vividly saw her rosy pink cheeks and droplets of water on her nose where the snow had melted. We then hit the bump. My reaction this time, as we came to a crashing halt, was, "Nobody touch me! Can't you see that I AM BROKEN?!"

Processing my dad's death was like being cracked open and all of my parts spilling out. I was foundationally broken and had absolutely no idea how to put myself back together. I felt like a literal Humpty Dumpty. My dad was the only person on this planet who saw me the way he did. I knew that no matter what I did, in his eyes, I was perfect. And I missed him so, so much.

What I missed the most was holding his hand. My dad had the softest hands. He always patted my hand when we were in the car driving together. It was his way of saying, "I love you," without words. If I were upset, he'd place his hand on mine and say, "Don't worry; things will get better." As he walked me down the aisle when I got married, I had one arm through his and held his hand with the other. As he lay in the hospital bed weeks before his passing, I held his hand for hours. In the days and months after he passed, I only wanted to feel his soft hand again—no words were needed because we had a language through our hearts.

The beauty of Divine Love is that it has the ability to transform even the deepest wound and offer the gift of grace. There have been so many tears while writing this chapter. However, as I reflect on all these experiences, I notice that these tears are no longer grieving his absence but rather profound gratitude for his presence and the lessons I learned from him throughout my life. My dad always treated me like I was a special gift, never to be taken for granted. I absolutely cannot believe how fortunate I am to have known this man and had the privilege of having him as my dad. I think of the miracles that brought me to this loving home, and I am humbled by this gift.

Throughout my dad's entire experience with ALS, he showed strength while facing adversity and an immense appreciation for the simple things. He didn't need words to convey his message. He showed his love and compassion through the kindness in his eyes and the joy in his smile every time I entered the room. He taught me to slow down. Have patience. And love fearlessly. This kind *gentle*man set an example to all by showing determination and humility, living with grace and peace each day, knowing that Spirit was on this journey with him.

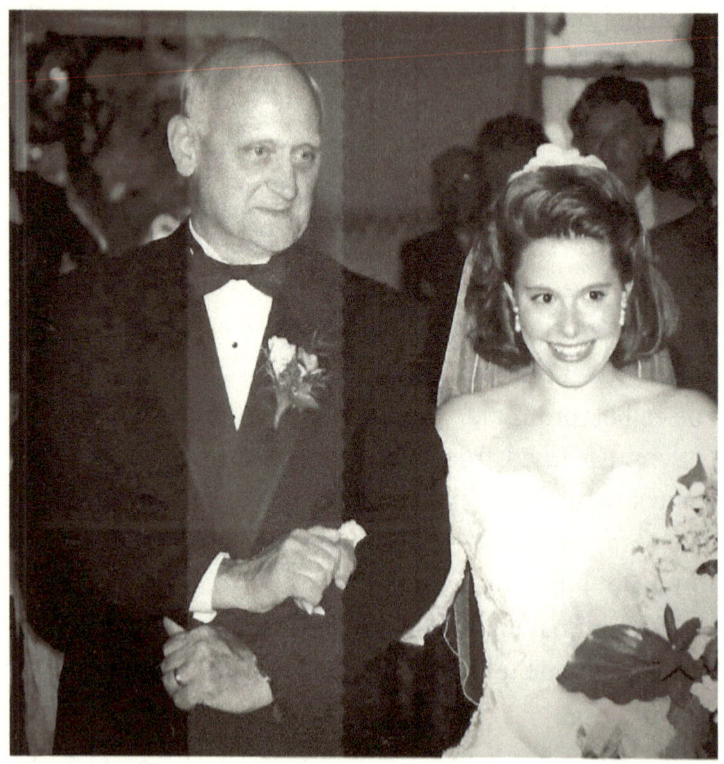

Help In Healing Through Divine Love

The key to awakening Divine Love within yourself is through finding grace for yourself and your journey. Grace means Divinely-Given Blessing. This blessing is an offering and a gift we, in union with Spirit, can give ourselves and each other at any time. Our heart is the space where this co-creation happens and is always open and awakened to heal any and all wounding. My healing process has taken many years. There is no time limit when it comes to healing and awakening the heart. Here are some suggestions to help you along your journey.

The key principles to applying the Sacred Truth of Divine Love to our human experience are:

- MOST IMPORTANTLY…Remember, the Divine essence of who you are is love.
- Know love for oneself and others.
- Understand compassion and empathy without pity.
- Give and receive forgiveness, acceptance, gratitude, and appreciation.
- Allow yourself time to grieve and also find peace.
- Speak to yourself with loving kindness and allow yourself to feel anything and everything without judgment.
- Find stillness and silence to hear the voice of your heart and Spirit.

- Practice self-compassion and forgiveness.
- Cultivate acceptance of your emotions. Every emotion is sacred and deserves to be heard and validated.
- Allow yourself time and space to process everything you are uncovering.
- Practice self-care.
- Take warm baths with rose water.
- Go on long walks.
- Practice slow flow or restorative yoga.
- Buy yourself some flowers or a beautiful plant to bring life into your home.
- Create a sacred space in your home for meditation and reflective time. Be sure to make it beautiful and comfortable.
- Try equal parts breathing (inhale, "I am love," exhale-gratitude).
- Speak with a trusted friend or counselor.

Divine Love Affirmation

"I am Divine Love. Through this Sacred Truth, I remember that the Light within my heart supersedes all fear and heals through unconditional love."

Journal Questions

- Write yourself a love letter. Find a special card or stationary and tell yourself all the things you appreciate and adore about yourself.
- What are some emotions that you have held close to your heart and would serve you to explore?
- Are there some old wounds that you have inherited from family or deep relationships that need exploring?
- Begin a gratitude journal. Express gratitude first thing every morning and last thing before bed. Begin with yourself and expand from there.
- Are you finding a balance between giving and receiving? Notice your patterns. Are you giving away more than you can afford to give? Do you feel that you are worthy of receiving love? If not, why not?
- Are you taking more than you feel you should be in relationships? When we are taking more than giving, the emotion of guilt often shows up.
- What are some nurturing words of wisdom you could share with your beautiful self?

Yoga & Meditation

Our yoga class and meditation are about awakening the heart and allowing it to speak. We will do various heart-opening postures, followed by time to listen, feel, and express anything that needs to surface. Divine Mother has a specific breathing exercise I will share in our meditation that bridges Spirit and the life force of the earth through the heart center. To access your classes, scan the QR code or visit the link.

https://bit.ly/3W3sueX

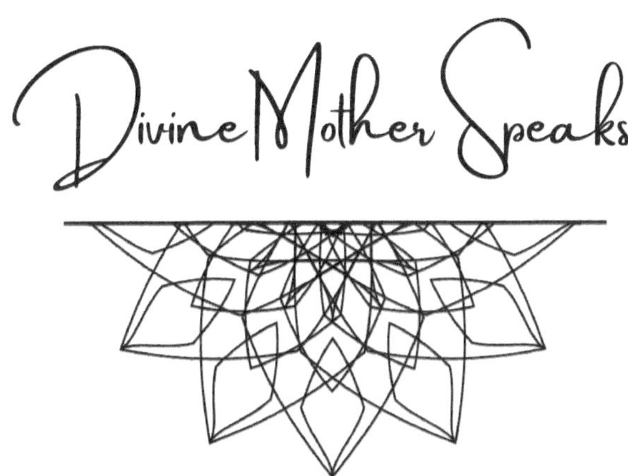

Divine Love

Beloved Ones,

You will never need to seek the external to find me because I live within your heart. You must simply fold into the core of your being and know that I am there.

My message is very simple. Be Love. Be Grace. Be Compassion. Be Joy.

"Be" means to embody the essence of Love, Grace, Compassion, and Joy. Think of the meaning of these words as an integral part of **who** you are rather than as an action you perform or an emotion you feel.

"Be" means that you encompass "The All That Is." It is remembering you **are** love. You **are** grace. You **are** compassion. You **are** joy. This is your birthright and is an expression of your Soul in its most illuminated form.

"Be" means that every cell in your body radiates with the Universal, Primordial Sound of Om—the purest and original vibration of Universal Love that beats within your heart. It is the vibration that the Universe receives and sends back with every breath. What I desire is for you to discover it within yourself. Once you embrace it, teach others how to discover it within themselves.

Yeshua came in to teach us this. He lived wholly through his altruistic heart and beamed love to and through the people. His gift was to see through a person and know their journey—no words need to be spoken. He could discern and extract the person's life experiences by allowing the entirety of his heart to read and feel the situation.

Yeshua loved everyone for who they were and how they showed up in each moment—never concerned for the person; instead, he embodied the ALL-knowing. And through his heart communication, he transformed any situation by casting a light, revealing that one's journey does not need to be shrouded in fear.

The heart knows your truth and will forever guide you in the most perfect and profound way.

Pause and Listen.

With Loving Kindness,

Divine Mother

PART III

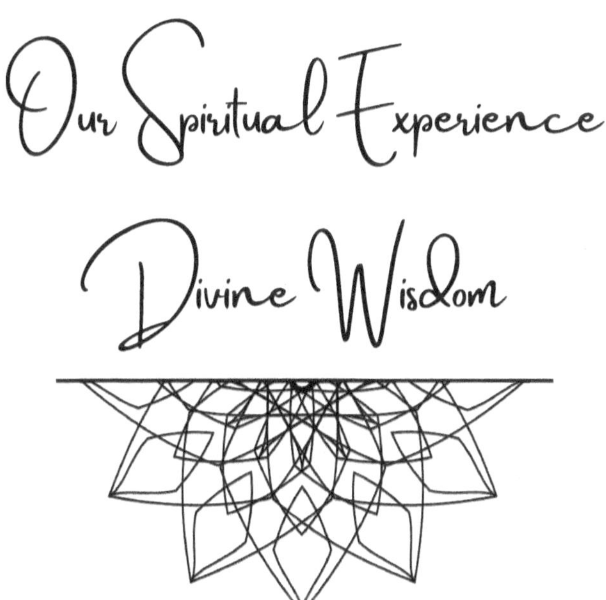

As we move into the final section of the book and upper chakras, I share from a more Spiritual and metaphysical perspective, including clairvoyant communication received in both conscious and dream states. The Fifth, Sixth, and Seventh Sacred Truths relate to one's etheric or Light body and are coupled with higher consciousness, truth, intuition, and purpose.

Chapter 5

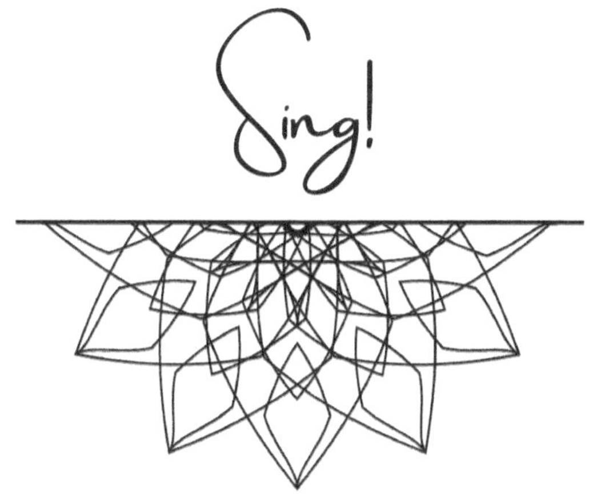

Fifth Sacred Truth
Divine Transformation

The purification aspect of Divine Transformation requires that you first awaken and empower your first four chakras or energy centers in order to fully access this Divine Channel. Each Sacred Truth and energy center builds upon the development, health, clarity, and openness of the prior Sacred Truths. This will increase your understanding and sensitivity, which will, in turn, gain you deeper access to the gifts of the more subtle upper chakras.

The Fifth Sacred Truth is Divine Transformation and the first of our Spiritual energy centers. It is the seat of truth; thus, every breath is an enlightened exchange of energy with the Divine. Our breath is the *vehicle* for Divine Light and Consciousness to enter and heal the body, mind, and Spirit. Divine Transformation calls us to become conscious of each breath as a gift because it is a living, sentient, integral reality.

Divine Transformation is a beautiful dance between Spirit and our soul, allowing your body to physically and Spiritually recreate, realign, and rejuvenate with every single breath. Think of your breath as the channel for Divine Light to move in and out of the body. Imagine the breath like a wave of light. As we breathe in, this wave of Light crests as it enters through the crown chakra at the top of the head. Riding on this wave of Light is the consciousness of Spirit/Universality. As the wave of Light moves through the body, it then folds into and infuses with our Soul/Individuality, and we become one. As we exhale, this wave of Light releases and returns back into the Universe, ensouled with our light, only to repeat itself on the next breath. Knowing that the breath is immersed in Divine Light, we can then begin to understand how Divine Transformation takes place within each respiration.

Now let's take it a step further. Consider the meditation from chapter four, in which I guided you through a pranayama (breath regulation) exercise that included the mantra A-U-M (Ah-Ooo-Om). Think of prana as light and mantra as form. When you combine the two, you create a hologram or matrix of light. As you breathe in light, you then become the light. As you hold it within the body, a transformation takes place, and you then ensoul the light––you integrate the qualities of Divine Light, and it heals the physical body and expands the Light body. Your soul is infused with the divinity and the life force of the Universe, which then attunes to your energy centers or chakras. As you breathe out, you return the perfection that is you back out to the Universe. So, imagine every being on this planet breathing the perfection of our life force in union with each other. If we focus on the Divine Transformation that takes place within each and every breath, how can we not heal ourselves and this planet?

When I work with clients in the healing room, I witness the wave of celestial Light that moves into them with every inhalation. Now, visualize every breath carrying millions of tiny particles of Divine Light. These particles of Light look like snowflakes catching the sun as they fall to the earth. I can see a spectrum of light or a rainbow ray captured within each snowflake. Every single breath we take draws in and then releases millions of these particles infused with Divine Light and Divine Love. They encapsulate every cell of our body. If we pause to witness and tap into this miracle that occurs approximately 22,000 times per day, we will be present in the healing that takes place with each transformative breath. It is a consistent reminder of our Divinity and perfection.

Divine Transformation aligns with our fifth chakra, Vishuddha (Vi-shoo-dha). The location is at the base of the neck, and the element is ether or space. Ether is the pure element through which sound travels. Space is all of the infinite, celestial universes which hold the primordial sound of Om—the original sound of the Universe. Think of the Om sound as a breath of pure Light and love vibrating from the infinite through every living thing on earth. This breath of Spirit then moves through every layer of the earth and grounds within the crystalline core of the earth. The earth's womb holds and intensifies this vibration of love, returning it back with the powerful sound of Om. This all-loving vibration encapsulates all living things on this planet and is then restored back to the Universe, only to repeat it again and again—just like a heartbeat. Do you recognize the similarities between the Om sound and your breath? There is a purification or cleansing that takes place with every breath, every beating of the heart, and every vibration of the Om.

"Sing!" is this chapter's title because singing is one of the purest vibrations of joy we can manifest through this powerful energy center. When we witness the ascendancy of the human voice singing, we see Spirit vibrating and transforming the singer and everyone in their presence. It is literally Spirit in action, as it communicates through the human body. This pure vibration is why we are so drawn to music! We can feel the vibration of Spirit and the angelic realms through the human voice. If you observe a singer, you can see that they are pulling from a source so deeply internal, transporting them to a higher dimension. Because their life force becomes so expansive, they have the ability to envelop the entire audience, thus holding the space and creating a container of Light for everyone in their presence to unite and transform into one powerful vibration of joy. Have you ever watched the television show *The Voice*? When someone's performance moves John Legend, he can hardly contain himself. He stands up, dances, arms in the air, eyes closed, and yells, "Sing!"

The dream I share here is a Divine Message that so beautifully articulates what I am describing.

My Channeled Dream—Sing!

In this dream, there was a beautiful woman singing on a mountaintop. She reminded me of Billie Eilish. She was young and full of pure expression, perfectly comfortable with herself and her gift. She had a powerful yet angelic voice. As she was singing on the mountaintop, she hit a note that no longer sounded human. The note she struck took on a life force of its own. Her voice turned into the purest tone—similar to a singing bowl's ever-expanding waves of vibration. It began to magnify as it projected outward. As she held the note, her voice grew and grew with intensity rather than weakened because she never ran out of breath. The resonance of this magnificent sound traveled and reverberated from one mountain top to the next, to the next, until it folded back into itself and began again.

There were judges present in my dream, almost like on the show *The Voice*. I was watching the singer as if I was watching it on television, but I was also there in person. I witnessed the intensity of her voice and of this mystical vibration encompassing all of humanity. I could see the vibration as much as I could hear it. I watched as this wave of sound connected with and actually created an energetic matrix or blueprint with everything in its path, whether it be human, animal, tree, stone, river, or ocean.

The vibration of her voice eventually ran through me. It felt like an internal explosion of light. Every cell in my body ignited with a euphoric sense of gratitude for the gift of life and the gift of complete presence. What I mean by presence is a feeling of perfect union and a sublime bond with all of humanity and every living thing on this planet and beyond. I was no longer separate from Spirit but a part of the whole that is Spirit. Everyone was a part of the whole, and each wave of Light reminded us of that truth.

In this dream, I realized that singer's voice *was* Spirit. It was the resonant sound of "The All That Is." This blessed singer became the primordial sound of Om-the original sound of the Universe. She was the vibration of Spirit, as was everything else in its presence.

The judges in my dream went wild. We were all immensely humbled as we witnessed and experienced Sacred Spirit channeling through this beautiful woman, expanding from mountaintop to mountaintop throughout the world and beyond.

Upon awakening from my dream, I felt a joy I have never known. I was being shown in this dream what it looks like and what it feels like to see Universality/Brahman (God/Spirit) when it joins in union with Individuality/Atman (humanity) and becomes one. I now *know* that I am the "oneness" of the Universe.

I received a gift that night. The veil was lifted for me, and I experienced Heaven and The All That Is. This, I promise—Heaven is not someplace up in the clouds. Heaven is us. Heaven is humanity. Heaven is knowing that *there is no separation* between our Creator, humanity, and all living things. This wasn't just a feeling or a dream. It. Was. Me. It is me. It is you. It is love in action—as a vibration of the whole. My "beingness," your "beingness," is love. And—love is Spirit.

As I went back to sleep, I sent out a prayer of gratitude for this experience. The response I received was:

The singer is you, the voice is you, the mountain is you, and…it is everyone and everything. Wake up, everyone, and be that voice. Be the essence of your pure love vibration. Let every thought, every word, every feeling, every action, and every deed be anchored in Divine Love. Then speak, sing, hum your truth to the world.

The Gift of Divine Transformation Through Self-Expression

The gift in Divine Transformation is two-fold. It is in our breath and also in our words. The fifth chakra is also the seat of communication and self-expression. When we live in alignment with truth and speak our truth, every word we say is also infused with the resonance of Divine Love. Our words create a vibration and become a hologram of light. We literally ensoul our thoughts into words when we find alignment to truth—truth being love, honesty, and integrity. When the intention of our words is love, they heal us. When the intention is malice, they harm us.

Because thoughts hold a vibration and a life force, just as strongly as if they become words, they birth ideas into existence. The more attention we give to them, the stronger the vibration and ability for them to manifest into reality. The more we can connect Divine Love with self-expression, whether through thoughts or words, the higher the frequency and vibration we send out into the world.

Where the fourth chakra is the bridge between our human and Spiritual experiences, the fifth chakra is the bridge between Divine Love (fourth chakra) and Divine Wisdom (sixth chakra). When we find the purity of love and the clarity of wisdom in our fifth chakra, our communication is crystal clear. We are able to speak our truth and also receive the truth with the highest of intentions. We understand the difference between "chatting" and honestly communicating our needs, desires, and heartfelt feelings.

When living in truth, we do not take words personally from another as we can see and filter out the difference between truth and projection. Rather than negatively reacting to another's comments, we can discern the situation without making assumptions, own our responsibility in the exchange, offer compassion, offer or request forgiveness, and release the rest. When you know you are going to have a difficult conversation, begin by infusing each and every exchange with Divine Love and Wisdom and notice the difference in your communication.

I'd love to break this down by describing an exchange I had with a friend that unfortunately went sideways. I'd like to precede this with one thought—texting and email exchanges are challenging modes of communication. Words, along with their intentions, are often lost in translation.

So this exchange began with a text message from my friend asking how I was doing. I responded that I was doing well and asked if she was working that day. The response I received was sharp and did not match the tone of our previous messages. Confused by her response, I asked what she meant. After not receiving an answer, I circled back the next day to check in. She suggested that we meet in person to clear the air. This confused me even more, but I agreed.

We hit another hiccup as we tried to find a location for our conversation. I decided to call and find out what was upsetting her. To be clear, neither of us is wrong because we each have different life experiences we are bringing into this exchange. In our conversation, she accused me of various malicious intentions. I had no idea where these feelings came from because she had never expressed them. The more questions I asked, the more heated the conversation became. Her words and tone felt accusatory, and I began to feel bullied. I requested that we hang up so I could sort through everything she said.

I needed to pause and separate myself from this experience by looking at the exchange as an observer rather than a participant. I decided to take a forest walk and asked Spirit to guide me through the exchange, help me find clarity in what my friend was expressing, and gain a clearer perspective on my feelings and intentions. I needed to release all attachments to my earthly experiences, such as being bullied as a teen.

As I was out for my walk, I received another snappy response from my friend. So I sent her a prayer of love, and I thought to my egoic self, *This is her issue, not mine.* But…the problem was, I still didn't feel good about it. I was *not* sitting in a vibration that was love and above, so I had a negative attachment to our interaction.

So, let's unpack this and find the truth in this experience versus the belief this interaction was triggering.

The truth is…

Something in what I said triggered something negative in her.

The truth is…

After reflection, I know in my heart that my comment and the words I chose had no ill intention.

The truth is…

Her response did indeed trigger something in me.

Pause…If I felt nothing from my friend's response, I would have no attachment to the situation. But I did feel something that wasn't pleasant, so I am now attached to the lower vibration of our exchange, bringing mine down as well. In order to get back to a place of neutrality with this exchange, I *get to* figure out why her responses bothered me and what belief she triggered in me that brought me down.

I know this sounds kind of silly, and you might be thinking, *Just forget about it and get on with your day.* However, we as human beings have become very fluent in stuffing down our emotions and getting on with our day, thinking these emotions will just go away. This is the reason my friend and I were at an impasse in the first place. There were clearly things that she had been feeling and never shared with me.

The truth is…

Our bodies store everything unless we can bring it back to a neutral vibration. The bonus is—we can actually transform and integrate our experiences back into a higher vibration. To be able to find neutrality, I needed to find compassion for both of us.

The truth for me in this interaction is…

I was bullied very badly throughout junior high, and her accusations began to feel like bullying and were doing damage.

The truth is…

I still have some work to do on my feelings of self-worth. In other words, it's okay if someone is mad at me or misinterprets my words. It doesn't make me or them a lesser person. I don't have to *fix* this interaction and convince anyone of my intentions to prove my worth.

In short, I am choosing not to honor the belief that "I am not worthy enough to be spoken to with respect," and instead am pausing to recognize that this dear friend of mine is simply working through some of her own hurt and is expressing that through her communication.

As I went through each accusation, I asked to see my truth in the exchange and be *completely honest* with myself about my most genuine intentions. My communication is far from perfect, but after returning from my walk, my heart and my truth knew that in this exchange, there was nothing loaded or ill-intended in any of my words—past or present. Obviously, something in my language triggered a negative response, so I reached out to her and apologized, being clear there was no ill intent.

Unfortunately, this did not help the situation and, in fact, made it worse. After this last interaction, I decided that I needed to step back from this friendship, allowing us both some time and space. This was a big step and quite healing for me to walk away. I feel resolved and at peace by taking the time to pause, reflect, discern, and, more importantly, offer myself grace in this situation, knowing my truth in our exchange.

As I get older, I recognize that it feels much better to accept responsibility in a disagreement and then own it, resolve it, and release it. Believe me; countless times, I insisted I was right and projected my righteous feelings onto someone else. We project to protect ourselves because of unresolved fear and discomfort with vulnerability. It isn't easy to look at our attachments and vulnerabilities and then own them. But in the long run, it is transformative and healing as it brings us back into alignment and our truth.

The truth is…

Neither my friend nor I was wrong in the exchange. We were just out of alignment. The root of our miscommunication came from each of us looking at the exchange through the lens of our individual life experiences and beliefs. Rather than going around and around, sometimes it is okay to walk away and allow some breathing room.

The truth is…

We find alignment and live in our truth when we see and communicate through the lens of Divine Love and Wisdom rather than fear.

The Gift of Divine Transformation Through Our Breath.

The gift in our breath impacts every part of us physically and Spiritually. There are so many fun facts about conscious breathing that support our physical body. Deep breathing decreases stress and increases calm. When we're stressed, the body releases the "stress hormone" called cortisol. Deep breathing slows the heart rate and allows more oxygen to enter the bloodstream, which then communicates to the nervous system that you are safe. Deep breathing releases endorphins which calm the body and help to relieve pain. It also stimulates the lymphatic system, which helps to release toxins from the body. Fully oxygenated blood carries and absorbs nutrients and vitamins more efficiently. The more oxygen that is in our blood means better organ function, better energy, and stamina. Deep breathing tells your muscles to relax, allowing your blood vessels to dilate. This improves circulation and lowers blood pressure. As you can see, so much goodness comes from mindful breathing, and it is such a simple thing to do.

Energetically, healing through our breath happens with each inhalation. As I stated earlier, every single breath ushers in millions of what I call *Spirit particles* or particles of light. I utilize breath and the *Spirit particles* in healing during my meditation time. When I am in meditation, I practice pranayama (mindful breathing). First, I take an internal view and witness my body as if I were on a tour of my insides. With my eyes closed, I can feel the subtleties of my body's wisdom and language. I then focus on the areas calling to me and attune to my breath. I can now feel the life force of each breath as it enters the chakra pillar and direct it where I need it to go. My breath feels like a pulsing wave as it enters my body. I harness the wave and begin to release all that is no longer serving me.

Help in Healing—Self-Expression

Because thoughts hold a vibration and a life force, just as strongly as if they become words, they birth ideas into existence. The more attention we give to them, the stronger the vibration and the more ability they have to manifest into reality. The more we can connect Divine Love with self-expression, whether through thoughts or words, the higher the frequency and vibration we send out into the world.

When we are out of alignment with our thoughts and words, it shows up as gossip, aggressive speech, unfiltered, non-discerning expression, nervous chatter, and an inability to listen and see others through a lens of love. Close your eyes and visualize what a vibration without love looks like. It's chaotic, disconnected, contaminated, and dense—the polar opposite of the singer I was just describing. This is why pause and reflection are so important. We are able to catch our thoughts, words, and actions before they manifest into something we truly do not desire.

If you find yourself in a disagreement or simply do not feel seen or heard, take a moment to breathe into your beautiful body. This helps to ground and re-center yourself. Feel yourself filling with Divine Light and Love. Lift yourself above the situation and look at it as an observer. What is your responsibility in it, and what is not? Own what is yours. Tend to what is yours. Heal what is yours. Release what is not by finding compassion and grace.

Help In Healing—The Breath

When I think about Divine Transformation, I am reminded of the balance between our inhales and exhales, giving and receiving, our universal self unifying with our individual self. Each and every breath has the potential to heal and rejuvenate the body and reconnect it with our soul.

In my yoga and meditation classes, as well as in the healing room, I assist my clients in finding healing through breath. I begin by having them sit in presence. I allow them time and space to find stillness, observe and feel the companionship of Spirit within, notice the subtleties of Light swirling about their body, and feel the Divine Existence that is them. I ask them to take a moment to honor their perfection and, finally, welcome communication with their body's wisdom. Next, I have them begin to notice the quality of their breath. I ask, "Is it entering your body with short, quick chest breaths? Can you begin to lengthen them into longer breaths by counting them out to 4, 6, or 8 beats? Can you fill your lungs and empty your lungs?"

172

The important part of pranayama, or breath control, is not only filling and emptying the lungs but also holding and retaining the breath. Visualize all of the beautiful rainbow ray *Spirit particles* floating into the body. By holding the breath to your comfort, you allow these particles to integrate into your cells, thus beginning your healing process. This healing can be physical, emotional, and Spiritual. As you become more fluent with controlled breathing, you will begin to feel the vibration of the breath, as I was describing. You can then direct the breath like a cloud of light into the areas that need your attention and slowly feel the shift and transformation taking place.

If I am in discomfort, whether it be emotional or physical, I visualize breathing in a ribbon of golden light into the area of discomfort. I then envision tying a bow around the area, moving on to each area of unease within my body until all have been acknowledged and tended to. I speak lovingly to my body and ask for it to receive the healing light. I call in my angels and Spirit to assist in this healing. I then go around and untie each ribbon one at a time, imagining that whatever the burden, let it be transformed, released, and reset. Pulling the ribbon out of my body, I allow the burden and distress to dissipate. I finish with some full-body breaths, giving gratitude for the miracle that is me and reminding myself of my perfection. This meditation has been added to the *Stand In Your Truth* YouTube playlist.

Divine Transformation Affirmation

"I am the Light of Divine Transformation and self-expression. Through this truth, I know I have the ability to transform because within each breath is the Light of Spirit, and every word I speak holds the resonance of love and compassion."

Journaling Questions

In reading this book, I fully encourage you to take time to unpack your experiences, no matter how big or small. What beliefs do you hold that create emotions not based in love?

• Your thoughts take on a life force. These thoughts are the beginning stages of manifestation. That holds a lot of power. Even feelings and unspoken words have a positive or negative vibration.

•How do you speak to yourself?

•What does your internal dialogue look like? What does it feel like?

•Where are the negative loops that keep you stuck?

•Is there a loving mantra you can create for yourself when you find yourself becoming negative? My mantra is, "I am love."

•Journal about at least one aspect of yourself you find beautiful.

•Do you take things personally and begin to spiral when a conversation does not go smoothly?

•What beliefs do you attach to these exchanges?

•Are you speaking to yourself and others through the lens of love?

•Do you recognize when your egoic mind steps in and derails a conversation?

•If we lack self-worth, we are afraid to be seen or heard and often just go along with others. Do you feel worthy of being listened to?

•This pattern also shows up by keeping secrets. What thoughts and feelings have you kept hidden? Can you begin to let them out by journaling about them? Are you afraid to be honest with yourself about your thoughts and beliefs?

•After doing the breathing exercise I shared through the meditation link, how did this make your body feel?

•As you partake in this breathing exercise, what is coming forward for you?

•Do you feel emotional or physical discomfort as you are releasing through the breathing exercise?

•Can you trace it back to its origin and begin to heal it?

•How does your body feel when you allow it to breathe deeply?

•How did this make your Spirit feel?

Yoga & Meditation

This yoga class will focus on slow fluid movements, with steady cleansing breaths. It will be a time of clearing emotional clutter and finding healing through the breath. The meditation practice will include breath (prana) and sound (mantra) to activate and cleanse all of the energy centers. To access your classes, scan the QR code or visit the link.

https://bit.ly/3W3sueX

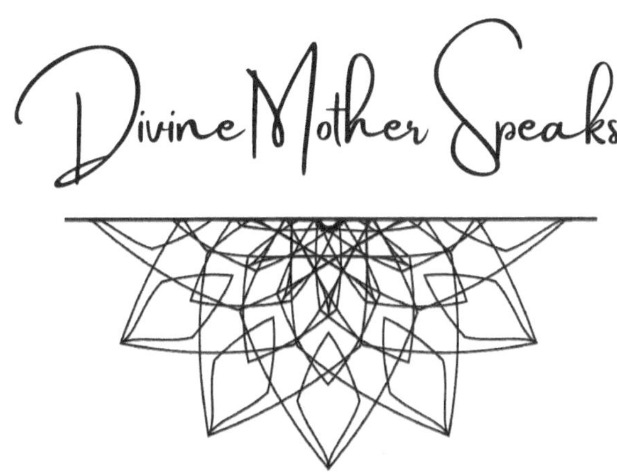

Divine Transformation

Beloved Ones,

May all creation sing!

Imagine the transformation when all creation sings in union, liberated from suffering, embracing the Light shining within you as one being with the Divine.

Did you know that your chakras sing? When living fully in alignment with the Spirit, each chakra manifests a beautiful grid of light that acts as an antenna, attracting more transformative healing light. All the colors of the rainbow glow and hum within your chakra pillar. They vibrate with the most angelic sound as each chakra finds its etheric frequency.

It's a symphony of light and sound proliferating as the Universe responds with tranquility. The only word to describe it is sacred.

With Loving Kindness,

Divine Mother

Chapter 6

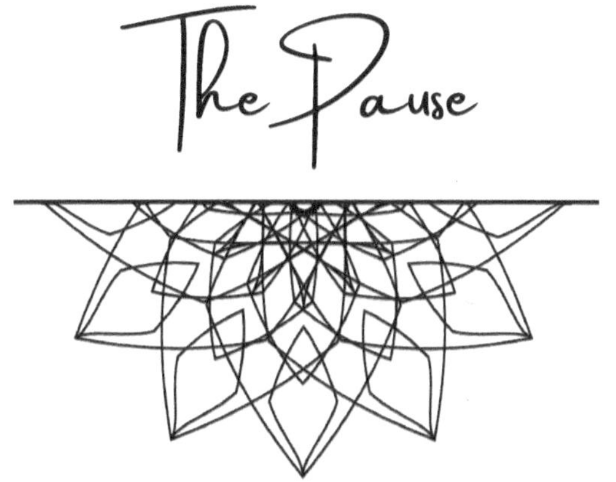

Sixth Sacred Truth
Divine Wisdom

"Divine Wisdom is about the process of renewal, expansion, and becoming consciously aware and awakened." –BT

As we continue to explore our Sacred Truths, Divine Wisdom is where we transcend the duality of looking at ourselves as human beings or Spiritual beings. The truth is there is no separation between the two. We are not separate from Spirit, nor are we separate from each other. The Sixth Sacred Truth is to maintain higher conscious recognition. In other words, remember who you are as a Divine Being. It is here we gain our second sight that turns us inward rather than to the external world. Our second sight is not seeing through our physical eyes but through an internal gaze grounded in divinity. We are able to use this second sight to discern and step fully into what we *know* vs. what we believe by illuminating the truth in all things.

Divine Wisdom intends to take on a higher, expanded consciousness, recognition, and intuition. The idea is to leave the egoic mind and humble yourself to become a true vessel for this Divine Perception. This means relinquishing all limiting beliefs about yourself and recognizing that you are indeed a Spiritual being. Divine Wisdom aspires to activate and maintain these levels of awakening, reminding us that with every breath, we are not satisfied with where we are but must move beyond, releasing structures in our life that keep us passive rather than illuminated.

The seat of Divine Wisdom lies within the sixth chakra, the Ajna (Aahj-nyaa) center. This energy center is located between the physical eyes, along the browbone, and regulates truth, self-evaluation, intellectual abilities, and emotional intelligence. The element of the Ajna center is Light and is associated with the illumination of all things. The frequency of the Ajna center vibrates that of unitive consciousness, oneness, infinite expansion, and Divine Understanding. The physical manifestation of the third eye is the pineal gland, located in the midbrain. The pineal gland has received much attention for its mystical qualities because it is the seat of communication between our enlightened being, the soul, and our physical being, the body.

The sixth chakra relates to our Divine Perception and expanding wisdom. It goes beyond the physical senses into the realm of subtle energies, such as our gifts of second sight, like…

Clairvoyance (Divine Guidance through internal imagery, an ability to see auras, energy, apparitions, and dreams). *Clairsentience* (Divine Guidance through feelings and emotions). *Clairaudience* (Divine Guidance through an internal voice). And *Claircognizance* (Divinely Guided thoughts). As you awaken to Divine Wisdom, there is no longer a filter on your past, your expectations, or your judgment because you can see them with sacred clarity. Even when our ego wants to resist, Divine Wisdom draws us to what is in our best interest.

Divine Wisdom teaches us that we are never separate from Spirit, even when we step out of alignment with our thoughts and actions. Divine Wisdom is infinitely expansive because it is your connection and union with Spirit and with each other. You *know* that there is no separation, even though you are in a human body, living an earthly life. Stepping into Divine Wisdom means surrendering the ego and all the beliefs you have subscribed to throughout your life. The way to know that something is a belief is that it doesn't allow you to grow and, in fact, makes you feel smaller.

Most of us came into a human body with the veil lowered. When we awaken our gifts in Divine Wisdom, we develop the ability to lift the veil and see that Heaven is within us and around us at all times. It is the thread that weaves us all together. Think of a newborn baby. This sweet, perfect human knows nothing about shame. All this baby desires is to be loved. And in exchange, returns that love. You were once and still are that perfect human. If this sounds hard to believe, consider this. Much of what happened between then and now have been life experiences in which your inner knowingness of your perfection has been trained out of you.

There's a quote I love by Wavy Gravy, the Woodstock poet/philosopher, "We're all just Bozos on a bus making our way through life." Isn't this the truth? We are all beautiful Spiritual beings, living and navigating our human experience together. You may feel as if you came in blind, without any sort of instruction guide or roadmap, but in actuality, you did. It is your Divine Wisdom. This is your way of navigating the world with an internal guidance by listening to the wisdom of the heart. You can see the journey not as it appears, but how it feels. Divine Wisdom asks us to step back and observe our attachments to situations and sort through the cluttered emotions based on past experiences and learned behaviors to see the truth. The truth holds no fear or negative vibrations because it is grounded in love. This may mean going back and exploring our foundational beliefs.

Take a minute to close your eyes and listen to what your heart has to say about it. Not what you have been taught, but what your heart is expressing. If the feelings coming up are filled with shame, guilt, or fear, these are just experiences that are surfacing and beliefs to which you have agreed. Gently allow yourself to unpack these feelings and know that it is okay to feel them. It is also okay to slowly examine where these feelings began. This is exactly what I do in my healing sessions. My clients and I unpack, explore, and unearth these beliefs until we get to the root cause of the shame, guilt, anxiety, fear, and any other emotion that is lower than love. We find that somewhere in their life, they were taught to feel this way based on another's beliefs that were simply passed down to them. As we awaken into our Divine Wisdom, we can rebuild our sacred vessel, weaving it together with the Light of Spirit. We're here to navigate this world together as best we can. And I believe the best way to do that is by tapping into your inner Divine Wisdom.

How do we step into and awaken our Divine Wisdom? The first and most important way to tap into your internal guidance system is through pausing, finding silence and stillness. It is the only way our Divine Guidance can be heard. You must put down your electronic devices, turn off the TV and radio, and deeply get to know yourself—not just your earthly self but, more importantly, your soul and your inner wisdom. I promise you that it always has and always will continue to enlighten your way if you simply quiet the mind and listen to its subtle voice.

The Gift in Divine Wisdom

There are many ways to receive Divine Wisdom. It just takes practice, patience, pause, and trust. The gift in this chapter is what Divine Mother asks of each of us: to pause. Our work right now is not in the ego, constantly "doing" and separating us from Source through constant distractions from our true purpose. Instead, we are being guided to allow space to just be. To heal ourselves and this beautiful earth, we must be still and return to our authentic selves because we are so much more than our egoic beliefs. Stillness allows us to breathe and remember who we are as Divine Beings.

Part of this journey is seeing humanity as a whole rather than as separate, splintered parts. Yes, we live our lives and have what appear to be individual experiences. However, our individual experiences continually intersect and impact that of the whole. Our life force is more vital when we understand that everything we do impacts everyone and everything—including the earth. Each individual vibration, whether high or low, feeds into the communal vibration of the universe. Our truth is *we are one* unified life force that ebbs and flows in a sea of Divine Light.

When our energy aligns to heal ourselves, it aligns with that of the Divine Mother to heal our planet. Our inner and outer worlds are one. There is no separation. The late Senator Paul Wellstone articulated this beautifully when he said, "We all do better when we all do better." An excellent example of this is *Ubuntu*. Ubuntu is an ancient African word. Roughly translated, it means "humanity towards others." I learned about Ubuntu philosophy when I came across a story about an anthropologist proposing a game to some tribal children in Africa. The story describes how he placed a basket of fruit or *treats* near a tree and had the kids stand a short distance away. He told the children that the first to reach the basket of fruit would be able to have the entire basket. Here's the beauty in this story. After he said, "Go!" rather than racing towards the basket individually, the children joined hands and ran together. Once they reached the tree, they divided the fruit equally amongst themselves. When asked why they chose to run together, they answered, "Ubuntu." One child said, "How can one be happy with the entire basket when the rest have nothing." Ubuntu, "I am because we are," is a universal bond and *the gift* we share that connects us all. This is co-creation at its best!

"Ubuntu means love, truth, peace, happiness, eternal optimism, and inner goodness. Ubuntu is the essence of a human being, the divine spark of goodness inherent within each being." –Eddy Kenzo

As we explore the Sixth and Seventh Sacred Truths, I will discuss healing through this truth and wisdom in addition to attaining this wisdom.

How to Develop Your Second Sight, Divine Wisdom

1. Remember Who You Are

A vital part of Divine Wisdom is remembering who you are outside of this fleshy body. Remembering who you are is seeing yourself as a Divine being and welcoming the influence of Spirit in all that you do. Divine Wisdom reminds us that there is no separation between the Light that surrounds us and the Light that we are. This is the foundation for the phrase, "I am that I am," or "So Ham," which means "I am of Spirit, and Spirit is of me."

When you remember who you are, you experience the wisdom to act thoughtfully and without judgment, while also being able to override fearful thoughts. You find confidence and neutrality in your decisions because they are Divinely Inspired and without attachment. Your inner voice is active and available because you have confidence in your intuition. This helps you feel motivated and inspired because you see everything clearly.

2.   Co-Create Your Life

Spirit is a part of everything. As I have mentioned throughout this chapter, you are *one* with the Creator, NOT separate. Pause and take a moment to consider where in your life you are floundering. You may feel that no matter what you do, you cannot seem to find your way through. The egoic mind chatter just keeps getting louder while also making you feel smaller. Spirit asks us to pause and observe the situation. Scope out and witness your thoughts and actions.

Are you loving into the experience? Are you asking for Divine Assistance and co-creating? I often find with my clients that they pray and pray and pray but see no changes. Remember, we are co-creating. Praying is only one-half of the relationship. Are you allowing enough silence and stillness to see or understand the answer to your prayer? Co-creation means that we are working together. It's a giving and receiving of energy and light. It has to go both ways by offering up your prayers and then pausing in reflection to receive the answer. It means pulling back from our impulse to "do something" and "trusting" that, with reflection, stillness, and silence, a solution will come that illuminates your path. It also means that the solution may not come the way you envisioned it.

3. Be the Observer of Your Dreams

The magic in the dream state is that your ego and analytical brain are on pause. The truth can come through without any intervention from the conscious mind. Dreams tell a story about how you authentically feel and what your heart desires. The trick is to put on your detective hat and decode their message. More importantly, dreams also allow us to receive Divine Information.

Some of my most profound messages from the other side have come to me in a dream state. There are specific dreams that I *know* I am channeling information from the other side and am guided to write them down immediately. I keep a journal by my bed, and many nights I have been dragged from my slumber to get up and write. When I awake in the morning, I am so happy I took the time to do so because of the intricate details captured immediately after the dream that otherwise would have been lost had I gone back to sleep. I also know that if I don't get up and write, I will keep myself awake anyway, going over these details in my head, hoping to remember them in the morning. In addition to the dream from chapter five, here are a couple more examples of channeled dreams with profound insight.

The Road Less Traveled

I remember a dream I had when I owned my yoga studio. I have always been an independent contractor, working for myself. When I opened my yoga studio, I wore every hat, from managing staff and clients to marketing, IT, teaching, doing my healing work, event planning, and even unclogging toilets. The list goes on and on. I often referred to my experience owning a small business as feeling like I was "pushing a boulder up a hill." There was never a time that I could just sit back and relax for fear this giant boulder would roll back down and crush me. It was a 24/7 undertaking. This experience continually stretched my limits and challenged every belief about what was possible.

This particular dream came to me shortly after my dad passed away from ALS, while also expanding the studio into a newer, larger space. In this dream, I was standing on the side of a steep mountain. My Uncle Chris was standing there with me. Uncle Chris was a very tall man with somewhat menacing eyebrows, a BIG voice, and an even bigger personality. He reminded me of John Wayne because he grew up as a cowboy on a ranch in South Dakota. He had giant hands and wore a big turquoise ring and cowboy boots. There was definitely a gentle side to him; however, there was also a don't-poke-the-bear side that I instinctively knew not to mess with.

So in this dream, my uncle and I were standing on a mountainside. As I looked around the landscape, I saw a very smooth, paved road contrasted with an incredibly steep, rocky, treacherous-looking path. Each of these routes led to the top of the mountain. He looked at me with a steely gaze and pointed sternly toward the rocky path. It felt clear to me at the time that he was foretelling my life's journey. When my ego and I woke up that morning, I remember thinking, *Oh great! My life is going to be rocky, unpredictable, and difficult.* This is exactly how I felt as I owned the studio. I interpreted the dream this way because this was the *belief* I was carrying.

I often thought about this dream. As the years passed and I grew more and more in tune with my Divine Wisdom, a different voice came forward. This voice reminded me of my dream and asked me to reconsider my interpretation. This voice said, "Is there another way you can look at this dream because we believe you missed its meaning? Instead of looking at the path as precarious, thinking it symbolized an omen of challenge and difficulty, could you shift perspective and consider that Uncle Chris was suggesting you will be 'taking the road less traveled' instead?"

By taking the road less traveled, this path empowered you to move slowly and thoughtfully, noticing and appreciating every single step forward. This path allowed you the opportunity to pause, reflect, and feel every part of your journey rather than speeding to the top and missing out on everything. This path enabled you to face challenges, sit with these challenges, learn from them, grow, adapt, adjust, succeed, then take another step. This path was a masterclass in understanding and exceeding your beliefs and expectations about your potential. This path blessed you with time well spent as you genuinely got to know your clients and instructors, developing solid, heartfelt relationships. It allowed you to grow into the teacher and healer you are today. It taught you humility and also offered you the confidence to eventually leave all you knew as a studio owner, only to find a new and expanded purpose.

This Divine Wisdom shifted everything and awakened gratitude rather than frustration. I made it to the top of that mountain, and now I have a knowingness that no matter what the challenge or outcome, all is well in the end. I know that challenge and contrast expand our experience. It nudges us to trust in something beyond our human understanding and capabilities. One of my students offered an amazing analogy for pausing while facing life's challenges. She spoke about the knot in a tree branch where new branches are in the process of being formed. There's a pause in this process where the knot forms as the tree figures out which direction to send its shoots. Then, it looks for the *light*, shifts direction, and, voila, new growth happens.

I am certain that each and every one of you has a story about a challenge you faced or are currently facing in life.

194

One in which you *believed* you could not surpass your current experience. Divine Wisdom will continue to ask you to "Shift how you are looking at the situation and continually seek the potential in your journey." Life is like a kaleidoscope. There is no right or wrong way to approach our journey. Each shift of the scope brings about a new, unimagined, beautiful picture.

The Big Stage—
Ego vs. Co-Creating

This dream began with me walking amongst a crowd into a large stadium. Looking at the crowd, I thought to myself, *You all don't know this, but I am the one singing tonight.* I remember feeling two contrasting emotions. The first was pride because my ego was saying, "You are so special because you will be the one up on stage." The second was overwhelming love as my Divinity said, "Won't this be a special experience as you create a union with this crowd through your music and voice?" Both of these contrasting thoughts felt equally powerful.

As I was awaiting my call to go on stage, I suddenly realized I didn't know the words to even a single song. In a frenzy, I furiously began to write some partial lyrics on my hand. With ink all over my palm, I took the stage. As I approached the microphone, I could feel the love from the crowd (Spirit in action) and also the panic and fear (ego in action) from not knowing a complete song. I kept looking at my hand and then at the crowd. Before I uttered a sound, I abruptly woke up.

What is the wisdom hidden in this dream? The Divine Insight is two-fold, both leading back to pausing and co-creating. In the dream, I held an egoic belief that even though I was walking amongst the crowd, I was separate from them and somehow more special because I was performing. Spirit said, "Imagine how powerful the experience would be if you were in union with the crowd, co-creating by giving and receiving." Now take this lesson and apply it to anything in your life in which you feel you need to navigate alone. Spirit says, "You are never alone. Your Divine Wisdom is ever present and available for you to tap into. Your only job is to pause, ask in thought or prayer, step back, and allow the wisdom to come forward to co-create a solution and a path."

The second message was, "Rather than seeking the external for inspiration (i.e., the lyrics), you have something fool-proof: your Divine Inner Guidance. Get out of your head and out of your way. Pause, listen, and allow Spirit to speak through you. When you tap into Source, you tap into the Universe's infinite wisdom." I have found this to be true as I teach a yoga class. My best classes are the ones that I intuit as I go. Yes, it makes me a bit anxious to walk into a class without a plan—but that is my ego saying, "What if you forget what you're doing?" I thrive in my teaching when I start the class slowly and observe everyone's energy. I navigate the postures and sequence based on what I feel and observe at that moment. It's a beautiful process of giving and receiving from my students, and it's all based on my Divine Wisdom rather than my ego.

Dreams are often the purest form of communication from the other side. I invite you to keep a journal beside your bed for 30 days. Upon awakening, take note and freewrite your first impressions and emotions about your dream because they reveal your most hidden feelings and beliefs. I also encourage you to take a pen and highlight portions of the dream that stand out. These images, impressions, and feelings are your most significant clues into what Divine Wisdom is communicating. If at first the meaning isn't clear, go back to reflect further another time. It is often then that we truly understand the meaning sent to us in our dreams.

Symbolism in dreams, such as animals, numbers, flying, falling, your childhood home, running away, or being pregnant, are examples of recurring dreams that help to decode your dream's meaning. For example, I often dream of owls. Owls appearing in dreams represent change, transformation, hidden knowledge, wisdom, and Spiritual evolution.

Recurring dreams are also an amazing form of Divine Wisdom's communication. One of my recurring dreams has a tiger loose in my neighborhood. I quickly shut all the doors and windows, only to remember that one of my children or pets is still outside. Inevitably, I cannot wrangle them to safety. This anxiety dream is my cue to release, surrender, and call in Divine Support for help in whatever may be going on in my life that is causing distress. The magic in dreams is that our inner guidance reveals things that our conscious mind may not want or be ready to address.

4. Soul Writing

Another way to hear the voice of your inner wisdom is through soul writing. Soul writing is sitting down with your journal and asking Spirit, "What do I need to know today?" I like to begin and end my day doing this. If I'm in a challenging situation, I ask, "What do I need to know about this situation?" At first, you may find that you continually challenge the messages you receive by going into your analytical brain.

The analytical brain will want to start fixing whatever you are asking about rather than allow time and space for clarity and for your situation to unfold. I still ask myself, *Is this my ego talking to me, or is a higher consciousness intervening?* The answer usually lies in how I feel about the answer. So I encourage you to ask your question, listen to the answer, and feel into the response. As I've said earlier, it is critical to be honest with yourself. Your heart knows the truth. If you're reactive, it usually means that your sweet ego is chiming in. Don't judge yourself. Just sit with the reaction and ask more questions about the origin of this reaction. Then write about it. Remember,

Divine Wisdom is expansive. Egoic thoughts are filled with structure, limitations, and fear.

5.   There's Magic in the Pause

If you're someone who always needs to have music or the TV on in the background, start slowly by turning it off. Daily periods of silence are the only way to hear your voice of Divine Wisdom. I find silence in many different ways. Some days, I absolutely love to sit on my meditation cushion, practicing pranayama, calling in Divine Mother, and listening to her response. I definitely recommend trying this because it can be the purest way to hear the voice of Spirit. It feels daunting to many, so I suggest setting a timer and beginning with just ten minutes a day, slowly increasing the time. Meditation is a disciplined practice but also offers great rewards. Yes, seated meditation is one way, but certainly not the only way. People often tell me they can't get themselves to do that. Understood. My advice is, then, don't. Begin your journey into silence another way. There are many ways to be silent and communicate with your inner wisdom without sitting on a meditation pillow.

I sometimes prefer to lie down on my yoga mat. This often puts me in an altered state. I know you are probably saying, "You mean to sleep?" And, yes, sometimes I fall into a sweet, brief cat nap. This tells me that my body needed a little rest. However, I often find myself somewhere in between a wake/sleep state. I call this my "download" time and often get some of the most profound information at these times.

The gift of silence can come from a moving meditation like a forest walk or run, digging in the garden, petting the dog, swimming in a lake, or standing outside in the rain. A friend told me she finds her Zen time while washing the dishes. The idea is to find peace, quiet, and the ability to still the mind, breathe deeply, calm the body, and listen to its wisdom. As I said before, the body never lies. What is your beautiful body desperately trying to translate for you? Find your place of Zen and listen.

6.   Hit Unsubscribe

What I mean by hitting unsubscribe is to quit accepting and agreeing to all the limiting beliefs you have been carrying around with you. It's truly a matter of cleaning house and clearing all the clutter in your inbox/brain/ego. First, notice how your thoughts and beliefs have made you feel throughout your life. Begin to pull back all of the layers of beliefs until you get to a feeling of expanded awareness. Expanded awareness means being completely honest with yourself. You become the observer of the experience or belief and release attachment. When I finally step into expanded awareness, there is no place to hide because the truth is staring me in the face. I no longer need to bury my feelings or pretend they aren't there. In these times, I feel the support from Spirit asking me to listen gently. It may not be what I want to hear or feel, but there is something so liberating when I finally allow it in.

The truth allows for emotional release, and it feels like I just put my bag of boulders on the ground and can move forward without all the weighted beliefs. Whenever something deep within my heart peacefully requests me to surrender, I know I will be freed from attachments and awaken to something greater. Truth frees up space for goodness to grow again.

Divine Wisdom Affirmation

"I am the Light of Divine Wisdom. Through this Sacred Truth, I remember I have an all-knowing, internal guidance, and sacred awareness at all times."

Journal Questions

• Do you find that you are indecisive? If so, what is the root of your indecision?

• Can you tap into your inner wisdom to help?

• Do you feel stuck with no vision for yourself? Write down your fears about moving forward.

•Do you feel lost on your Spiritual path or life purpose? Take a minute to daydream and write down what truly inspires you. You may need to dig back into your childhood.

•Do you feel you are living entirely in a fantasy or daydream state and are uncomfortable living your daily life? What makes you uncomfortable? What in your life are you avoiding?

• Do you find yourself overriding your heart's desires with analytical thinking?

• How much of your time is spent absorbed in mind chatter?

• How much of this mind chatter has been integrated into your beliefs?

• Do you often get stuck in a loop, as in "going down the rabbit hole" or feeling disempowered based on your thoughts?

• Do you feel open to a higher power?

• Do you recognize when you are given Divine Wisdom? How does it come in for you? Write about how it feels.

• Do you recognize your ability to co-create with your Divine Wisdom?

• Can you feel the emotional difference between your intuition and your intellect?

• Does your intuition reveal a more profound level of truth?

• What beliefs and attitudes in yourself would you like to change?

• Can you commit to making those changes?

• Do you procrastinate taking action even though you recognize this change would benefit your life?

• Can you identify your reasons or fears for not taking action?

Yoga & Meditation

This chapter's yoga class will guide you into the pause by exploring nurturing, restorative, yin style postures. With eyes closed, I'll ask questions during the practice about what is being communicated via your body's wisdom and also through the heart. The accompanying meditation takes you through a breathing exercise to activate and balance this powerful energy center. You are prompted to tap into your internal voice, listening to these pearls of Divine Wisdom to help you find ease in co-creating your life. To access your classes, scan the QR code or visit the link.

https://bit.ly/3W3sueX

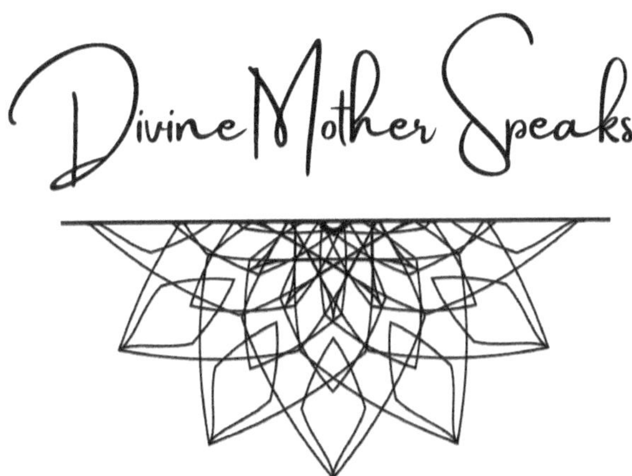

Divine Wisdom

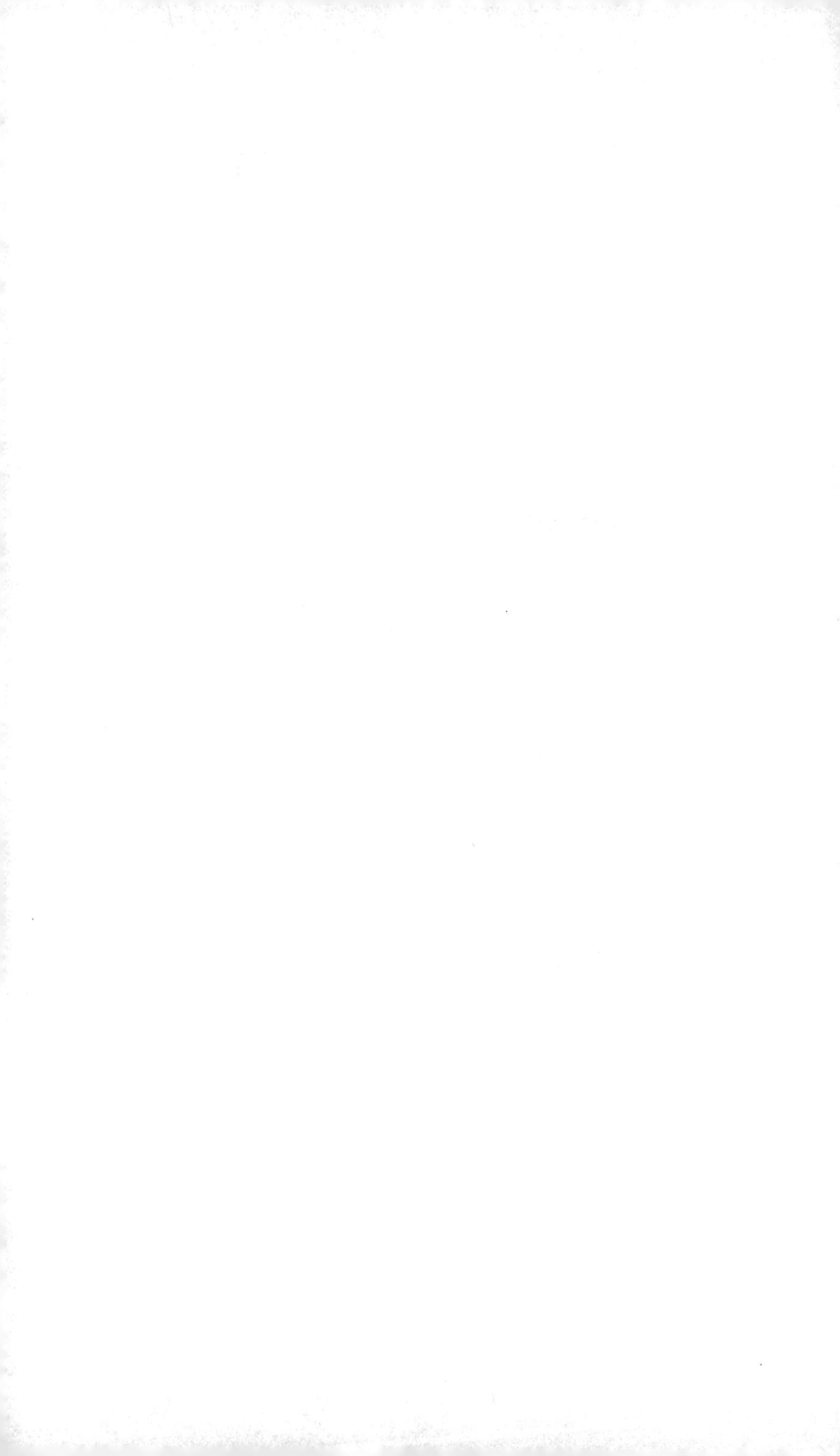

Beloved Ones,

What does it mean to exist in the pause—To be still?—To be silent?—To be aware?—To take notice? Understanding the pause means to live deeply in the rhythm of life while allowing for undisturbed serenity. The pause is the perfect compliment to rhythm.

Take a moment. Breathe. Observe. Be honest with yourself. Are you synchronizing with the rhythm of life or in opposition to it? Are you enhancing the rhythm or creating contrast? Are you in harmony or dissonance? Are you living in truth?

The pause provides time and space to get deeply rooted, stable, and connected with oneself. Only then are you able to make choices based on profound, truthful observations rather than chaotic responses or reactions.

Balance pause with action, pause with prayer, pause with an inner knowingness and expectation that you have been seen, you have been heard, and you are profoundly loved. Trust the silence and the stillness. Recognize that the Universe is knitting an alignment through the stillness. Meet that alignment and be still.

Stillness is a focal point at which one takes notice of the movement of life, offering the ability to honestly observe all the moving parts and best understand one's place within the rhythm. Stillness reveals the truth.

Release all judgment of yourself. Be forgiving with your thoughts, tender with your heart, and gentle with your sweet, miraculous body. Think softer. Feel softer. Be softer. Slow down and rest. Reflect. Feel compassion. Feel blessed. Know your beauty from the inside. Adore yourself as I adore you.

Pause. Breathe. Love.

With Loving Kindness,

Divine Mother

Chapter 7

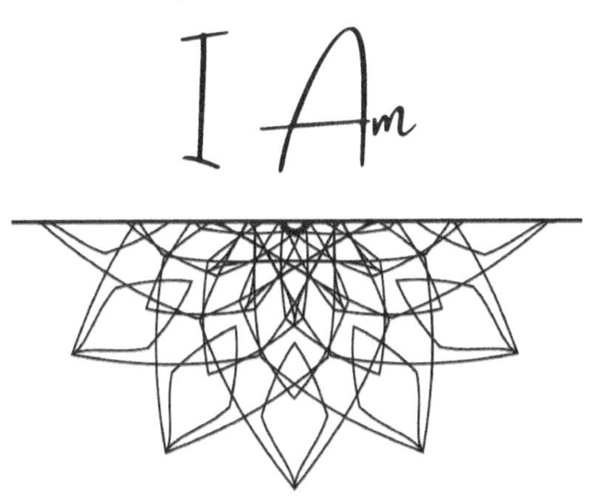

Seventh Sacred Truth
Divine Light

The crown chakra is the gateway to Divine Consciousness. The sacred Divine Intention for your crown chakra is to hold yourself in a *God state* at all times. This Divine Truth reminds us that we are not separate from each other, as we learned in the previous chapter. Living in a God state and integrating this Sacred Truth means knowing we are also not separate from Spirit. Rather, we are one with Spirit. Spirit is not only within us but *is* us. We are one with each other, the Universe, and Spirit—*and* we are love.

The location of the crown chakra/Sahasrara (Suh-hus-raa-ruh) is at the top of your head. It is often referred to as 1,000 petals opening up to the Heavens. My observation of the crown chakra is a spiraling vortex of Light moving downward into the top of one's head. The crown chakra is the center of Divine Inspiration, Wisdom, Unity, and our connection to All That Is.

Just above the crown chakra is your oversoul or, in Sanskrit, the Antahkarana (On-ta-kar-on-uh). Your oversoul, which sits about 18 inches above our human head, is where we have transcended human reality. The oversoul is a radiant orb of Light that contains your entire existence—past, present, and future. The oversoul maintains flawless coherence to our Divinity and is the blueprint of your perfection.

The Brahmadvara (Bra-mahd-var-uh) is the gateway to our crown chakra and is the receiver of Divine Light. Think of Spirit as a giant power source of Divine Light, sending out the energy of unconditional love. Now imagine that infinite cords of light are coming from this one main source, Spirit. This network of chords plugs into each crown chakra and reverberates through every human being and every living thing on this planet. The Divine Light then grounds into the earth and down to its crystalline core—only to return up through the earth, through our life force, and back to its source.

The Gift of Holding Oneself in a God State & Remembering The All That Is

Standing in *truth* is knowing that it is impossible to be separate from Spirit and each other. We have a human body and an etheric or Light body. Everything in the human body comprises energy—every atom, molecule, cell, and tissue. Even our thought processes are composed of energy. As a healer, I see this energy show up as clouds, sparkles, and orbs of light. Our Light and the life force that runs through our physical and Light body are all interconnected with every living thing on this planet in addition to Spirit.

Our human experience can sometimes feel very isolating, and it's easy to question why we feel this way if we are Spirit in a body. The answer is, at that moment, we are not *standing in our truth* and are out of alignment. Living in presence and in the Light calls for constant attunement. It is certainly not something I feel every day, all day. But the gift of presence is that my heart knows this unbreakable connection, and when I am able to tap fully into my heart, I find my way back home to Spirit.

While in meditation, I received this imagery to better explain our oneness with Spirit. Imagine the vast ocean. If you were to take a bucket of water from the ocean, would the water in the bucket not still hold the ocean? Now imagine several buckets of water being pulled from the ocean. They may seem separate because they are in individual containers, but if you were to pour all of the buckets of water back into the ocean, they, too, would become the ocean once again. Now visualize that the ocean is Spirit, and the bucket is our human body. Since our bodies are energetic containers of light, not only your body but that of everyone on earth is a beautiful, sacred vessel, holding the essence of Spirit within. We are not separate; rather, we are a part of the whole, resonating the essence of Spirit throughout the Universe.

The gift in Divine Light is to know nothing but pure bliss. It is to remember that all things vibrate in love, and we are an integral part of this vibration. It is to release all structures that minimize our existence. It is to live as one beating heart of Divine Love. The following experience describes a night I was spiraling with anxiety in my egoic mind. I was praying for some sort of relief when suddenly, I was lifted out of my body to be shown what it means to be in a *God state*. This was my experience.

Here I sit, awake again in the middle of the night. It is 3 a.m., and my anxiety is beginning to rise. In a couple of days, I will be taking my daughter to the Netherlands for school. She's not just going for a semester but her entire undergraduate program. I've gone through college goodbyes before with my older two, and I know the drill. The anticipation of it is far worse than the actual goodbye. There's something more uncomfortable about this goodbye because she is the last one to leave the nest. We developed a fun adult relationship while she took a gap year due to Covid. When all is said and done, I know I have raised a smart, independent young woman who is more than ready to take on the world. And yet my heart aches that she will be so far away in a location I have only seen in pictures.

What is it about waking in the middle of the night that stirs up such magnified discomfort? I'm in awe of the contrast. One minute, I am peacefully sleeping, then the next, I am fully awake, going down the rabbit hole as my emotions take a stronghold over me. As usual, I send up a prayer to my guides, guardians, angels, all beings of light, Divine Mother, Great Spirit, and truly anyone who is up and will listen. I'm asking for help pulling me out of my self-made misery as I let go and release my daughter into the world, praying she will be safe. I have learned as a parent that from the moment our children are born, our job is a continual lesson in letting go. It begins the second they cut the umbilical cord until the time one of us crosses back to the other side.

On this night, as I pray, a sense of calm washes over me. I feel a sacred hand on my heart. Gently, my Spirit begins to rise out of my body, and I elevate above my bed, above my home, and above the earth. I don't feel separate from my body, but I am also not attached to it either. And yet, I am able to see and feel everything. I have this soft awareness that I have become everything.

I am the air. I am breath. I am my body. I am the earth, the trees, the sky, the sea. I am all of this. I Am All That Is.

I have no fear. I am gifted with a peaceful yet profound understanding that I am one with everything. I always have been since the beginning of time. I am the I am.

In this moment, I have a keen awareness of just being and only knowing the now. The anticipation of a future or memory of a past is not relevant or even possible. Time is irrelevant. There is only now.

I feel weightless. My beingness feels like floating in calm water or an early morning mist that is softly rising. It appears like the colors of dawn. My physical body is now expanded into infinity. My consciousness is also infinite. I feel everything. I am awakened to all beings everywhere because they are now a part of me. I have expanded beyond human understanding. The best way I can describe it is that it feels like a view of how Spirit observes us. Every emotion melds into one experience, and that experience is love. There's an indescribable sense of ease because everything just is. Judgment and fear do not exist. There's no achieving. There's no better or worse. All expectation is released. There isn't a time or space for fear. It is the All That Is, and the All That Is is perfect unity or a perfect unitive consciousness grounded in pure love.

This experience does not express euphoria either because that would mean there has to be an opposite or opposing emotion. It feels like I just arrived into blissful acceptance and will always be in this constant state. I no longer have to strive to be anything else because there is a sustained knowingness that all is well.

During my experience, I was also able to scope out and observe all of the souls on earth currently inhabiting human bodies. These souls were bouncing around, bumping into and intertwining within each other's experiences. Being a witness to humanity while also being a part of humanity makes me feel like it's no wonder souls are waiting for a turn to jump into a body. I was in awe as I witnessed the wisdom humans gain by navigating the contrast of emotions in just one single moment. The beauty and insight we receive while on earth allow us to have such rich, tactile, and experiential understandings. As humans, we can feel, touch, laugh, and cry. We can

216

hold someone and also be held. It's so profound to hold a loved one's hand or be wrapped up in a beautiful embrace with heart pressed against heart. That is a pure, human expression of Spirit.

We as humans seem to experience our lives as being separate and individuated from each other, but that isn't the truth. Living in a human body makes us feel like I am me and you are you—that our encounters are divided. This is an illusion. Authentically, we are vibrational beings. We cannot help but intersect with each other at all times. You and I are one within Spirit. We all meld into one consciousness.

When we feel contrast in our lives, it is simply an expression of feeling different, divided, or apart from the whole. We feel separate from each other—separate or detached from joy, love, or maybe abundance. For me, it's a feeling of being out of alignment and fragmented from my Source. It feels like I have stepped out of the Light and into the shadows of my ego.

The truth is, we always return back to ourselves, back to our oneness, back to center, back to our Divinity, and back into the light. Anything else is simply an illusion. We always are and always will be fully and unconditionally loved and connected to Spirit.

During this awareness of feeling The All That Is, there was only love. It was a constant. It was unconditional and inseparable. I was inseparable from my Divinity and the Divinity of everyone and everything.

This experience I am sharing with you only lasted a few minutes. As I have reflected on this over the days following, I have been trying to step back and simply witness my relationships with love as a mother, daughter, sister, friend, wife, and, most importantly, with myself.

Unconditional love is difficult to translate into human terms because of our fragile and oftentimes overpowering egoic selves. I believe we like to think that the love we know and understand in human relationships can be unconditional. But with the way society has conditioned us to look at and experience love, is it really? I would say the closest I have come to understanding unconditional love has been as a mother. I simply cannot fathom that anything would disrupt this bond and my love for my children. I am also blessed with an incredibly happy marriage. I loved him the first time I saw him. I even told my parents after our first date that I was going to marry this man. My mom responded that she said the exact same thing to my dad. We were engaged three months after we met and married within the year. Over 30 years later, I still deeply trust in this love with my husband. I feel very secure and grounded in our relationship. I love being in love with him.

As much as I love this man, there are still variables that can upset this beautiful balance…because…as most of us have, I have been socially and generationally conditioned to look at love through the lens of emotion and action. If we must do something or be something or feel a certain way in order to give and receive love, this makes love a commodity. This makes love conditional. It is something that we must always tend to, or we believe it may go away.

The difference between my experience in this altered state and my earthly life with myself, my children, and my husband is that during this brief period, the veil was lifted, and I experienced a constant and unyielding vibration that I am safe because I AM LOVE—not lov•ed, but LOVE. And that vibration of being love is the difference between love as an action and the full integration of love as a part of my being. It removes all conditions and egoic illusions that one must do something in order to be loved.

The truth is that love is not a commodity. Love is not finite. Love is not an emotion or an expression. It is not something that is given and received. Simply put: LOVE IS WHO WE ARE. This means we cannot be separate from each other. We cannot be separate from our Divinity. Love is pure coherence with our Divinity and that of each and every living thing on our planet and beyond. This experience allowed me to fully explore and awaken to my oversoul and remember the perfection of humanity when we sit in alignment with the Divine.

So…I pose this question to you. Can you open your heart, your pure beingness, and wrap it around this truth? We absolutely must begin to view our experience here on earth through a different lens because we are united in everything as one unitive consciousness. Anything below the vibration of love is just an illusion we have chosen to subscribe to.

Today, I ask you to please, please remember who you are! Every thought, every word, every deed, and every action carries a vibration that impacts each other and our planet.

You are love! Sit in the vibration of love and feel what happens. It is absolutely magical and probably the most profound experience I have had in this lifetime!

After reading this, I encourage you to take a moment in silent meditation and enjoy the pause. Begin to slow your breath down, taking deeper inhales. Pause with your inhale, feeling the purest Divine Light expanding within every cell in your body. Then move into a slow, steady exhale, releasing the unconditional love-filled Light back to infinity. Continue to repeat until you feel yourself slipping into tranquility.

Before you return to your day, bring your hands to your heart for a moment. Begin a mantra with your slow, steady breath.

Start by saying, "I AM LOVE...I AM LOVE...I AM LOVE."

Move on to, "WE ARE LOVE...WE ARE LOVE...WE ARE LOVE."

Finish with, "WE ARE ONE...WE ARE ONE...WE ARE ONE."

Bring your prayer hands from your heart to your third eye center.

"May you have peace in your thoughts."

Bring your prayer hands to your lips.

"May you have peace in your words."

Bring your prayer hands back to your heart center.

"May you have peace in your heart and your actions."

Be love!

How to Awaken and Heal Through Divine Light

Now that we have arrived at the Seventh Sacred Truth, it is important to maintain coherence with all previous Sacred Truths.

The way I unify is through grounding breath. Just a reminder—our breath is the vehicle for Divine Light to enter the body an average of 22,000 times each day. With each breath are millions of rainbow ray Spirit particles lighting up our physical and Spiritual body. My hope is that with consistent practice on focused breathing, you will not only be able to see the Light as it enters your body but also feel its resonance and presence within. My clairvoyant gifts transformed as I became more proficient with my pranayama (breath work) practices.

The way to awaken to our truth of Divine Light is to integrate all seven truths into our Light Body and then into our Physical Body. Once we *know* and hold these truths within our heart rather than understanding them through our intellect, we are prepared to awaken to the *I am*—meaning, "I am of Spirit, and Spirit is of me."

I have a lovely practice that I would like to share with you that can help you with this process. It's called *The Seven Stages of Presence* and was passed on to me by my Spiritual teacher. The only way to become the Light is to create a Divine Vessel within our human body to hold the Light we seek (First Sacred Truth, Divine Manifestation). This practice is helpful because it is a reminder not only to our physical self but also to our Light body that we *are* the perfection of Spirit.

To begin, find a quiet place to be still and be silent. Take a moment to listen to the subtleties of your body's wisdom. Ask, "Is there anything I need to know in this moment?" Then calm the mind and sit in presence. Sitting in presence is not just feeling your purest love and Divinity within you; it's *becoming* this love. Sitting in presence is remembering who you are and knowing your perfection as a Divine Being—it's a conscious recognition that I am of Spirit, and Spirit is of me. It means that there never is nor has there ever been a separation from Spirit because we are one.

Sitting in presence feels as familiar as your own skin and the beating of your heart. It is not just visiting for a fleeting moment; it is an integral part of who you are. If you struggle with this, that is perfectly okay. That is why you are reading this book and doing this exercise—so that you open yourself up to receive the gift of Divine Presence and universal, unconditional love. I do not sit in presence at all times. However, through my meditation and pranayama practices, I know that I have the ability to tune into it. I hope to continue my Spiritual journey and elevate my vibration so I may live in this state at all times. The key is to eliminate distractions and be in the pause.

As with everything in the book, give yourself the grace to begin with baby steps. You can send up a prayer something like this —

"I may not feel your presence, but I am letting you know, Spirit, that I am opening my heart to the best of my ability at this moment. I am requesting to feel your compassion and love while learning to trust, feel safe, and be vulnerable. I am open to and desire to love myself and feel that I deserve to live in unconditional love."

Then just sit for a moment, breathe deeply, and be with your beautiful, perfect self.

Divine Light Affirmation

"I am Divine Light. Through this Sacred Truth, I am expanding my Light body and knowing my connection to all things."

The Seven Stages of Presence

In the exercise below, I am taking all of the Divine Affirmations and am integrating them with the breath for more integrated healing. It's important to speak these affirmations out loud. Remember that words carry a vibration, and hearing these affirmations help the truth to integrate and ground within your body.

Let's begin.

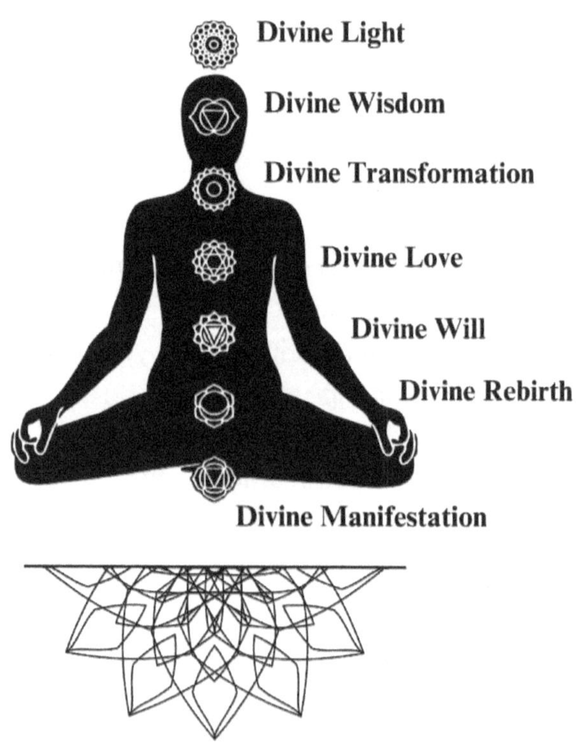

By breathing the Light from our oversoul (the magnificent orb of Light that sits about 18 inches above your head and holds the blueprint to your perfection) into the crown chakra (at the top of the head), then guiding it into the chakra pillar (located along the spine), and grounding this sacred Light into the earth, we create a continuum of all our conscious Sacred Intentions.

1. Sitting up or lying down with your spine straight, gently breathe into your crown chakra with a long, slow, steady breath through the nose. Pause and hold the breath in your body once your lungs are full. Slowly exhale through your nose. Then say, "I am Divine Light." It's important to say this out loud so the vibration of your words is not only heard but deeply felt. Repeat these steps three times to allow better integration of the Light. Finally, breathe from your crown chakra at the top of your head down to the first chakra at the tip of your tailbone. Again, breathe slowly through the nose. Pause and hold your breath. Gently exhale. In doing this, you are expanding your Light Body and feeling the connection to all things.

2. Following the same method as above, breathe into the sixth chakra (third eye), which is the space between your eyebrows along your brow bone. Pause and hold the breath. On the exhale, say, "I am the Light of Divine Loving Wisdom." This helps you remember that you have a higher, all-knowing, all-wise, all-

seeing awareness at all times. Please repeat this three times.

3. Breathe into your fifth chakra, located at the base of your neck. Pause and hold the breath. On the exhale, say, "I am the Light of Divine Transformation and self-expression." This reminds you that with every breath, you have the ability to transform, because within each breath is the Light of Spirit. Every word you speak holds the resonance of love and compassion. Please repeat this three times.

4. Breathe into your fourth chakra, in the center of your heart. Pause and hold the breath. On the exhale, say, "I am the Light of Divine Love." Remember that the Light and love within your heart supersedes all fear and heals through unconditional love. Please repeat this three times.

5. Breathe into your third chakra, located in the solar plexus/diaphragm. Pause and hold the breath. On the exhale, say, "I am the Light of Divine Will." The Light of Divine Will within me allows me to supersede my ego and surrender to the truth, thus allowing me to feel the beauty, bliss, and perfection in all things. Please repeat this three times.

6. Breathe into your second chakra, located just below the navel. Pause and hold the breath. On the exhale, say, "I am the Light of Divine Rebirth." Through this truth, I have all potential to transform, regenerate,

renew, and reawaken all things. Please repeat this three times.

7. Breathe into your first chakra, located at the tip of the tailbone. On the exhale, say, "I am the Light of Divine Manifestation." Through these truths, I have created a sacred vessel to hold this Light. It is completely grounded and integrated within both my Light body and physical body. All is love, and I require nothing else. "And so it is, and so it shall be." Please repeat this three times.

Journal Questions

- Do you feel a connection to a higher power? If not, what is the barrier preventing you from allowing this relationship?

- Do you feel like you have a Divine Purpose in this lifetime? What does your gift to the world look like? This does not need to be a grand gesture. Being an example of human kindness or a guardian of the earth and to all creatures, big and small, fulfills this purpose.

- How can you do more of what inspires you to continually seek and live in your purpose?

- Are there ways you can simplify your life so you live less in the distractions of the material world and more in your Divinity?

- How can you be of service to others?

- When and how can you incorporate daily silence, prayer, and meditation time?

- Do you seek Divine Guidance during meditation? Try asking, "What do I need to know?" And then pause to receive the answer.

- Do you feel you have received a response, and how does this response come to you?

- Are you open that this response may not be precisely what you asked for but may actually turn out to be better?

- Consider ending your meditation (prayer) time with gratitude.

- Do you have Spiritual truths that you live by? (We identify these truths because they are based in love.)

- Are you devoted to a particular Spiritual path? If not, do you feel the need to find one?

- Do you fear expanding your Spiritual path and creating a closer relationship with the Divine because of changes it might trigger in your life?

- Do you spend too much time in meditation and in the Spirit world, avoiding or not tending to your daily physical needs?

- Can you identify what is making you uncomfortable in your physical existence? What is it?

- What would bring more balance into your life?

Yoga & Meditation

The accompanying yoga class will blend the energies of yin and yang (feminine and masculine) postures, beginning with sun and moon salutes and ending in some lovely restorative poses. This practice brings balance and union to the body, mind, and Spirit. In our final meditation, I will guide you through *The Seven Stages of Presence,* ending with *The Circle of Light* exercise designed to unify all beings everywhere through the power of loving intention for our planet and all who inhabit this earth. To access your classes, scan the QR code or visit the link.

https://bit.ly/3W3sueX

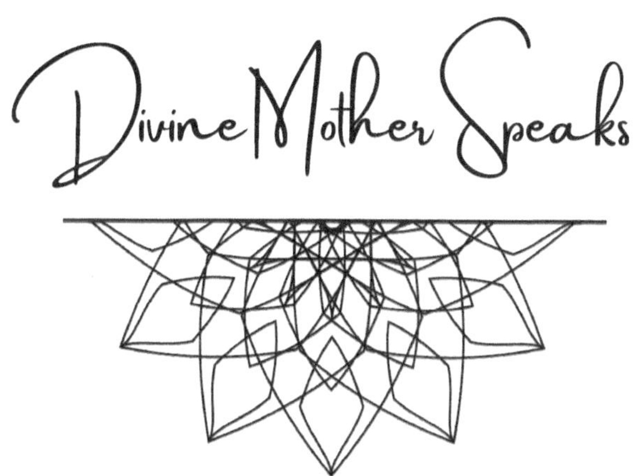

Divine Light

Beloved Ones,

Through my words, I am offering you a transmission of light. Feel the imagery. Allow it to penetrate and heal your precious body, mind, and Spirit. In doing this, you become The All That Is.

Please find a quiet place to sit and receive.

Imagine yourself standing on the edge of a cliff. You are dressed in a flowing garment of pure diamond-white light.

Now take a moment and envision the sky. It is the perfect balance between day and night. The sun is setting as the moon is coming up. Picture a full spectrum of brilliant colors in the sky as the first stars begin to appear.

The landscape beyond you is lush, filled with a myriad of trees, flowers, birds, butterflies, and waterfalls. The air is light and filled with the aroma of both flora and fauna. Feel the softest breeze gently touching your skin.

Listen to the sound of the waterfall in the distance and birds chirping their last song of the day.

The purest vibration of love softly moves in and out with each respiration and beating of your heart.

Gently release your arms down to your side and extend them out as if you are receiving the most precious blessing. Feel the light breath of air blowing against your face. Uncurl your fingers and open your hands as if you are allowing each and every burden to simply scatter in the wind.

As you are relinquishing your burdens, take care and be soft with yourself. Know that my love exists within you at all times, and I will assist you in this process.

Slowly feel your life force getting lighter but, at the same time, more potent because it is no longer encumbered with the weight of suffering.

Every part of you is now adorned with Divine Light. You are luminescent and weightless.

You are free. You are love. You are one with everything.

Now visualize yourself taking flight because you have become the All That Is. You are a part of everything, and everything is a part of you.

This is God State. This is Heaven. This resides within you always.

With Loving Kindness,

Divine Mother

To close out our journey through the Sacred Truths, I ask that you find a lovely card. Address it to yourself. Then sit in presence for a moment and write yourself a love letter. Write it as if your soul, the angels, Spirit, and Divine Mother are witnessing your innate beauty and perfection and are speaking directly to you. Find a special place to keep this letter and read it often.

Chapter 8

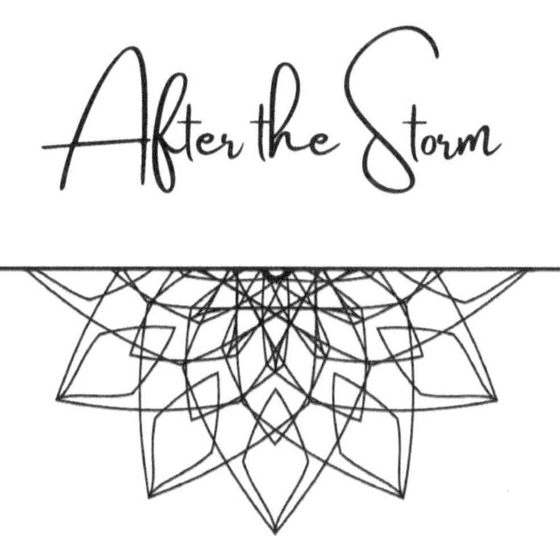

This chapter is named after one of my paintings, *After the Storm,* which is also the cover art for this book. A miracle is associated with this painting that relates directly to my dad. The title and the imagery of this painting are also a metaphor for this book. The thunderstorm represents the emotional and Spiritual struggles we, in our humanity, manage throughout our lives. Think of these struggles like a cloud of congestion held within the body. As we remember our innate wisdom and *Stand In Our Truth*, the clouds begin to clear, and the sky opens up, illuminating this blessed truth—we are perfect, Divine, sacred beings, living in the vastness of Divine Love.

Living in truth and Divine Love opens the door for miracles to happen because we are centered in the purest of alignment. In the following stories, I share some of the miracles that have blessed my life when I found alignment with Spirit.

Rainbows

Thunderstorms are a big part of our summer when you live in the Midwest. The day's heat builds, the wind picks up, and the sky gets dark as ominous clouds move in. The energy begins to electrify the air as lightning strikes. Everyone goes inside to hunker down as the storm pushes through. And then suddenly, all goes quiet. As the skies clear, the first thing you hear after the storm is raindrops trickling off the rooftops, and the birds begin to sing again.. There is a freshness to the air as the sun peeks through the clouds. And if you're really lucky, maybe you will see a rainbow.

My dad passed away on May 11th, 2011. I remember feeling the silence after he passed. I thought surely, with my clairvoyant gifts, I would immediately pick up the communication we had developed while he was in a body but couldn't speak. As a medium, I also get visitations from people who have crossed over all the time, so why would this be any different? But as the days and weeks passed, I couldn't find him anywhere. I couldn't feel his presence at all. It was as if he didn't exist any longer. I was the loneliest I had ever felt in my life. I remember being so angry at the silence. I could not understand why we must feel that much pain and such deep separation from our loved ones after they transition. It felt cruel. I was completely ungrounded and in a very dark place, trying to find a sense of normal in my life after the years of my dad's illness.

As I moved into summer, I began to speak regularly to my dad, even if I couldn't hear anything back. My birthday was coming up in late July, and I asked my dad if he could send me a rainbow for my first birthday without him. It could be our little wink of communication because rainbows will forever remind me of dancing in the living room to "Somewhere Over The Rainbow." Rainbows also remind me of miracles.

On the evening of my birthday, a big thunderstorm rolled in. I felt hopeful my dad was going to answer my birthday wish. My girls and I were driving home from dinner when the storm hit. Each of them was looking out a different car window for my rainbow. As the storm lightened, we stopped in the Target parking lot to scan the sky. The sun was setting as the clouds cleared, so I took a picture of the colorful sky. (That photo became the subject matter of my painting, *After the Storm)*. We kept looking, but the sun began to make its way to the horizon, and then it was gone. Sadly, there was no rainbow to be found. I told my dad, "It's okay. I know that was a big ask."

Since we were at Target, one of my daughters asked if we could go inside and look around. I agreed because who doesn't love a good Target run? As we got inside the store, everyone dispersed, and I waited near the front in the jewelry department. There was music playing. Suddenly, the music abruptly stopped mid-song. I was expecting someone to make some sort of announcement. I was *not* expecting what would happen next. A moment later—I kid you not—one verse from Judy Garland's original version of "Somewhere Over the Rainbow" played throughout Target. I looked at the woman standing next to me and yelled like a lunatic, "Did you hear that?!" (Think of the movie *Elf* after Will Ferrell just drank the entire bottle of soda.) The expression on her face was priceless. It was a mix of "Should I call security or just acknowledge and ignore the crazy lady screaming about the music?" I was absolutely elated and also so shocked that I couldn't even process the miracle that had just happened. As I write this today, it's still hard to believe it did.

The lesson I was reminded of through this miracle is that our special people who have crossed over are always around us. They hear every thought and prayer. They want to support us in any way possible. After my dad transitioned, I was living in a cloud of grief. So much so that I couldn't find him anywhere, but that doesn't mean he wasn't present, listening, and sending love. It was my work to raise my vibration and attune to his, not the other way around. I needed to find my alignment and stand in my truth. The truth is, there is no separation, whether someone is in a human body or a spirit body. My miracle came to me because, on my birthday, I found hope again. I had faith like a child and knew my dad was with me. And this is the key; I surrendered all expectations as to what, if anything, was going to happen. I matched my dad's vibration of Divine Love, and our synergy manifested this miracle. The beauty is that creating miracles is available to everyone. We must know they are possible, step out of the way, and allow them to come through the veil without holding expectations as to how they will show up.

My birthday miracle didn't stop there. I received a rainbow in the sky on my birthday for several consecutive years after this event. These occurrences eventually stopped because my heart had healed. I discovered I didn't need to see a rainbow to know he was there. I had established a stronger, more profound relationship than the one we had together on Earth. This doesn't mean that I don't still miss holding his sweet, soft hand, but I know one day, someday, I'll walk the rainbow bridge, and we will be reunited.

Pennies From Heaven

In the final days of my dad's life, some old neighborhood friends came to say goodbye to my dad. As they were leaving, the wife said to me, "Look for pennies from your dad. You know, pennies from Heaven." Pennies never really meant anything to me before. But I thought, well, okay, I'll watch for pennies.

After his transition, to my surprise, whenever I thought of my dad, a penny would randomly fall in front of me, or I'd see one on the street while walking. If I sent a prayer to him, asking for affirmation on something, the next thing I knew, I'd find a penny in my pocket. So pennies became a thing and another way he would communicate from the other side, letting me know he was there and listening.

Occasionally, I have dreams about my dad. During this particular dream, I was in northern Minnesota, staying in my favorite cabin on Lake Superior. In this dream, my dad laid out three pennies on a dark brown dirt path. At the end of the dream, I told him, "I'll follow you, Dad, don't worry, I'll follow you." And then I woke up. I got out of bed and went to sit in the front room to look out over the water, trying to make sense of it. I soon got distracted and went on with my morning, releasing all thoughts of the dream.

Later that day, my hubby, Joe, and I went for a hike on the Canadian border. Shortly after we got on the trail, I looked down at the dirt on the path and was reminded of my dream. I told Joe, "Oh yeah, I woke up from a dream this morning. My dad was laying pennies on a path. The path in my dream looked exactly like this one." A few moments later, as we were walking, I saw three pennies lined up on the path exactly as they appeared in my dream. I received the message that he would be walking the journey with me throughout my life, continuing to open my eyes to all the miracles around me. He asked me to keep my heart joyful and said, "All things are possible when we look at the world through the lens of a child."

Time for Me to Fly

It's been nearly three years since Tyler crossed. I came upon his memorial bench tonight while out for a walk along the river in downtown Stillwater. I could feel his spirit as I sat down. There was just a subtle, sweet sense of joy. As I was taking in the beautiful night air and view of the river, I could faintly hear the lyrics from a 1980s REO Speedwagon song, "Time For Me to Fly," playing at an outdoor restaurant.

Just like the miracle with my dad, I only heard this one verse—*"I know it hurts to say goodbye, but it's time for me to fly."* This verse began to play over and over in my head the day Tyler crossed and for months afterward. Like an earworm, I'd even wake up in the middle of the night, replaying this one lyric in my head. This verse made me think of him riding on his Harley, wind blowing his hair, wearing his cool headband and sunglasses, and just feeling free. Because of this, I requested that this song be played at his celebration of life.

As I sat on the bench processing what I was hearing, all of the emotions of losing Tyler came flooding back. I was hit with a massive wave of grief and guilt. I felt grief because I missed sitting by the river with him and guilt because my final goodbye, my final words were not, *I love you.* Because of that, I continue to live with such regret. In this moment, I feel as if I will forever wonder if my words or actions could have made a difference the night he accidentally overdosed. But even more than that, I missed the opportunity to remind that kid one last time that he is so so loved.

As I am writing this, Divine Mother is reminding me that no words are needed because, just like my dad, Tyler and I understood the sacred communication through our hearts. My heart knows this to be true, but right now, my mind and my ego are attached to the idea that I did not take any action the night before Tyler died by speaking the words, "I love you," or looking him in the eyes and hugging him. My ego is keeping me stuck in a lower vibration of self-condemnation. I hear the wisdom of Divine Mother, but in this moment, I do not feel it because another layer of grief is exposed, and I feel raw again.

After a night full of tears, my emotions have finally settled, and my heart is beginning to open. I am able to receive this miracle as a gift from Tyler, presented to me as a gentle nudge that I have more work to do. This was an invitation to dig deeper and find a more impassioned level of grace and forgiveness. Grief is such a mysterious emotion. You never know when and under what circumstance it will reveal itself, nor do you have any time limit on when it will subside.

So when I ask myself, "What do I need?" the answer is always, "Time." For me, grief is not something that can be fixed or talked through. There's nothing rational about it. The beauty in grief is that it is an incredible expression of love, yet at the same time, it feels like loss. But the truth is the person who crossed is not lost. We, the survivors, just can't find them because our pain clouds the view. When the heart finds its way through the pain, turning grief into gratitude, that is the point at which the healing can begin.

With all of my heart, I love you, Tyler.

The Sacred Heart

The final story I'll share is about Divine Mother. Hopefully, throughout the book, you have become familiar with the essence of Divine Mother, feeling her nurturing and compassionate, loving kindness coming through with each blessing.

Being raised in the Catholic church, Divine Mother has shown up for me as Mary, mother of Yeshua. She is known by her sacred heart and is identified symbolically through the rose. As I grew into my Spirituality and left the constructs of organized religion, I have known Divine Mother not simply as the Mother of God but as Mother Divine Herself—the Divine Feminine. I found a beautiful quote by Paramahansa Yogananda that articulates Her magnificence perfectly.

"Divine Mother is so beautiful. But remember, in Her higher manifestations, even that beauty is formless. She is in everything. Her Divine, compassionate love is expressed in the raindrops. Her beauty is reflected in the colors of the rainbow. She offers fresh hope to humanity with the rose-tinted clouds at dawn. Above all, be ever conscious of Her presence in your heart."

While preparing to write this book, I spent hours upon hours in meditation with Divine Mother. In my reflection, I was guided to go to a sacred shrine where apparitions of Divine Mother have occurred. As a result of these apparitions, several miracles have taken place for people who sat with Her, praying for healing. I had been there a few times and felt this would be a great way to align my Light and listen to Her wisdom.

Upon arrival, I got out my journal and found a comfortable place to sit in the sanctuary. I immediately began channeling pages and pages of wisdom. On this trip, I spent about ten hours sitting vigil, writing, and receiving over two days. Much of this shows up in the blessings concluding each chapter. After the second day, I felt complete, packed up my car, and headed home.

Upon returning home, I unloaded my belongings. As I picked up my suitcase, I saw a beautiful rose quartz heart sitting underneath it. I was taken aback because I had never owned a rose quartz heart, and the back seat was completely empty as I loaded my suitcase into it earlier in the day. I found myself trying to figure out some sort of reason this could have ended up in my car, but there was none to be found. As I sat holding this beautiful heart in my hand, the Light within it told me all I needed to know. My love for Divine Mother manifested another miracle. This was her gift to me and a reminder that she is ever present in my life and that of the world. I now use this sacred heart in my healing sessions, allowing my clients to hold it and feel its calming and nurturing vibration.

The Gift in Manifesting

When we are attuned to the Light and our Divinity, miracles happen. Remember that our very first sacred truth is Divine Manifestation. This truth is about creating a sacred vessel and foundation to hold the Light we wish to receive. I know that I was able to manifest these miracles because, in those moments, I found pure alignment. In each of my experiences with my dad, I felt such love for him and our relationship. I was filled with gratitude and could feel his presence within me regardless of how things were to manifest. The same is true for Divine Mother. As I sat in vigil over those two days, I just knew that the messages she gave me were sacred. I felt her life force moving through me like a wave of light-filled love and compassion.

What was shown to me through these experiences is that when we ask for some sort of communication or gift, it comes to fruition when we stay in alignment. We cannot attach to how it will show up. Attachment is our ego saying, "I know best." Divine Will says, "Surrender your attachments, and we will show you something so much greater than you ever imagined." I am still in awe that my dad was able to get ONE verse from Judy Garland's original "Somewhere Over the Rainbow" to play in the middle of a Target store! I could never, ever have imagined something so extraordinary.

Please know that I have experienced many lessons around manifestation. My ego and Divine Will have gone head to head many times over the years. I remember when I first learned about manifesting through the Law of Attraction. The idea of the Law of Attraction is that our vibration attracts a like vibration. My initiation into the Law of Attraction was applied to manifesting the home of my dreams. I'm a little embarrassed to share this, but it is the perfect example of how attachment to an outcome can get in the way of what you want to bring forward.

Many years ago, a contest on a home fix-it network gave away a "dream home" at the end of each season. The home given away for this particular season was in the Florida Keys. When I saw this, I thought, by hell or high water, I was going to win this home by applying my new knowledge of the Law of Attraction. The contest rules allowed you to enter your name once a day, every day until a week before the drawing—which I set my clock to. On top of that, I printed up images of every room in this dream house and put them in a scrapbook. I looked at these images daily, visualizing the joy of living in this home with my family. Full disclosure—this became somewhat of an unhealthy obsession. Though a bit concerned, my sweet hubby never said a word about my behavior.

At the time of this contest, it was the end of a long Minnesota winter. I was feeling very unsettled in my life and did not have clarity about my future. I was still working as a fashion stylist, living in the city. Although it was a fun career, it began to feel meaningless. I was craving purpose, expansion, nature, and more freedom. This contest felt like the answer to my prayers. As I meditated, daydreaming about my future home, I felt alive and excited about moving our sweet family of five to sunny Florida. As the drawing came closer, my excitement grew. On the night of the "big reveal," we all sat around the television with anticipation. Well, at least I was waiting with anticipation. The other family members were most likely there to support my soul-crushing reality when I did not receive a knock on my door telling me, "You are the winner!"

Needless to say, I did not win. I was disappointed, but as I went to bed that night, it was almost as if the fog had lifted, and I could see that this wasn't how the Law of Attraction and manifesting miracles work. My lesson was two-fold. I was obviously attached to an outcome, and this attachment pinched off any and all potential for manifestation. My view became so myopic, and I was solely fixated on this particular home. I squeezed the so-called bar of soap so tightly that it slipped out of my hands.

On the flip side, there was something in me during this time that had faith like a child. I learned that anything is possible by holding on to my childlike faith. Now I send up a prayer and allow Spirit to create the perfect gift. This is the true magic that results in miracles.

As I put this lesson into practice a few years later, I did manifest my dream home in a little river conservation community. The difference between this home and the "dream home" in Florida is that there is a sense of ease in this neighborhood and in my life. Every time I turn into our neighborhood, I feel like I am going to the cabin. I remember when we first moved in, a neighbor drove by and said, "Welcome to God's country." Everyone in this small community has the same appreciation for the simplicity of nature and the water. I am now living my purpose as a healer and am running my business from my home. All of my clients can feel the peaceful vibration as they take in their session. I am convinced that the solitude of nature is what allowed me to hear Divine Mother's wisdom and request to write this book. And writing this book has been the greatest work of my life so far.

Miracles can and do happen every day. Most people don't think to ask for them or become frustrated that these gifts from Heaven don't show up when and how they hoped. My message is simple: Our communication with Spirit is a giving and receiving between thought, prayer, reflection, and pause. Ask away for anything and everything your heart desires. But then pause and listen. Then listen further. Listen, listen, listen. If you want to hear and experience the response from the other side, you have to be in a place to receive it. As I said earlier, turn down the noise in your life. Flip off the television. Put down your smartphone. Drive in silence. Get out in nature. Take time to be soft with yourself and just breathe. This is the only way to hear the wisdom of your body and the wisdom of Divinity—as they are one and the same. After you've done all that, *trust* that your thoughts, feelings, and prayers have been received and are in the process of being answered in the best way possible. Get out of your own way and release expectations about how they will appear. That's the gift in a miracle: It's a surprise every time!

Ever since I was a kid, sitting in my *I Dream of Jeannie* pajamas, trying to blink myself into other realities, I believed in magic and miracles. You have to believe in miracles to create them. It isn't lost on me that one of the lines from the song "Somewhere Over the Rainbow" dares us to dream. I dare you to dream and dream big, just like you did as a child before all of your beliefs clouded your view. I challenge you to release all the reasons why something won't happen and, instead, expect great things to happen. It may not be exactly how you thought it would look, but in my case, it was so much better than what I ever imagined.

Journal Questions

- Think back throughout your life. What is something that you always wanted and you were actually able to manifest? How did it feel to bring this gift forward? How did you release beliefs and *know* you could do it?

- All manifestations must come from the heart. What is something that your heart truly desires? Write or pray about it. Ask Spirit for guidance. Trust that your intention has been heard and answered. Stay in a place of pause and silence in order to receive. Get out of the way and allow Spirit to present you with the perfect manifestation of your desire. Journal about the journey.

- Think about your daily routine. Are there ways you can remove distractions and find times of silence?

- Each day, write down any synchronicities you notice. Remember, synchronicities occur when your vibration matches that of something else. Manifesting miracles requires us to synchronize with the life force of the Divine and our loved ones on the other side.

Conclusion

Even though it may not always feel this way, it is a significant honor to live in a human body during this time in history. We are here as pioneers while the earth is experiencing immense changes due to our actions and those who came before us. Our purpose is to remember it is no longer possible to experience ourselves as separate from anything or anyone. When you *Stand In Your Truth* by integrating the Seven Sacred Truths, you can review your blueprint, recognize where the distortions lie, and change the sequence.

In other words, we need to *be love* by emanating love from the core of our existence. Each of us has a vital part to play in elevating the collective consciousness. And as we raise our vibration we create a new framework for the earth to heal itself and all lifeforms. Consciousness restores balance. And unless we ALL are free, none of us will be. This path aligns with our soul's purest journey.

To *Stand In Your Truth,* it is imperative to practice the Seven Sacred Truths and make them a part of your everyday reality. These intentions are an opportunity to recognize that this is a pure awakening of "The Self." In doing this, you enlighten yourself to its higher soul's recognition and remember your innate perfection *because* you are love.

Collectively, as one vibration rises, we all rise.

In love and light! Suzy

Please visit Suzy's website to book a healing session and for further information.

www.suzyschaakyoga.com

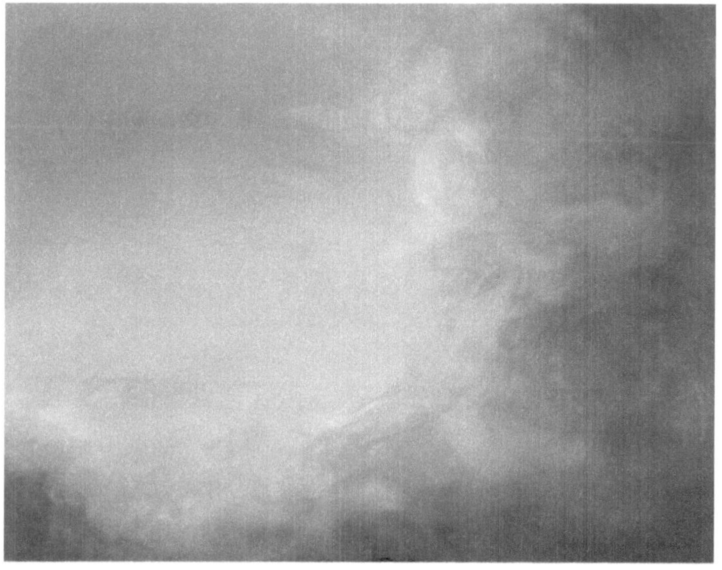

To purchase a print of *After The Storm* or other pieces by Suzy, scan the QR code or visit the link.

https://www.etsy.com/shop/SuzySchaak

www.ingramcontent.com/pod-product-compliance
Lightning Source LLC
Chambersburg PA
CBHW032012150726
47990CB00005B/1936